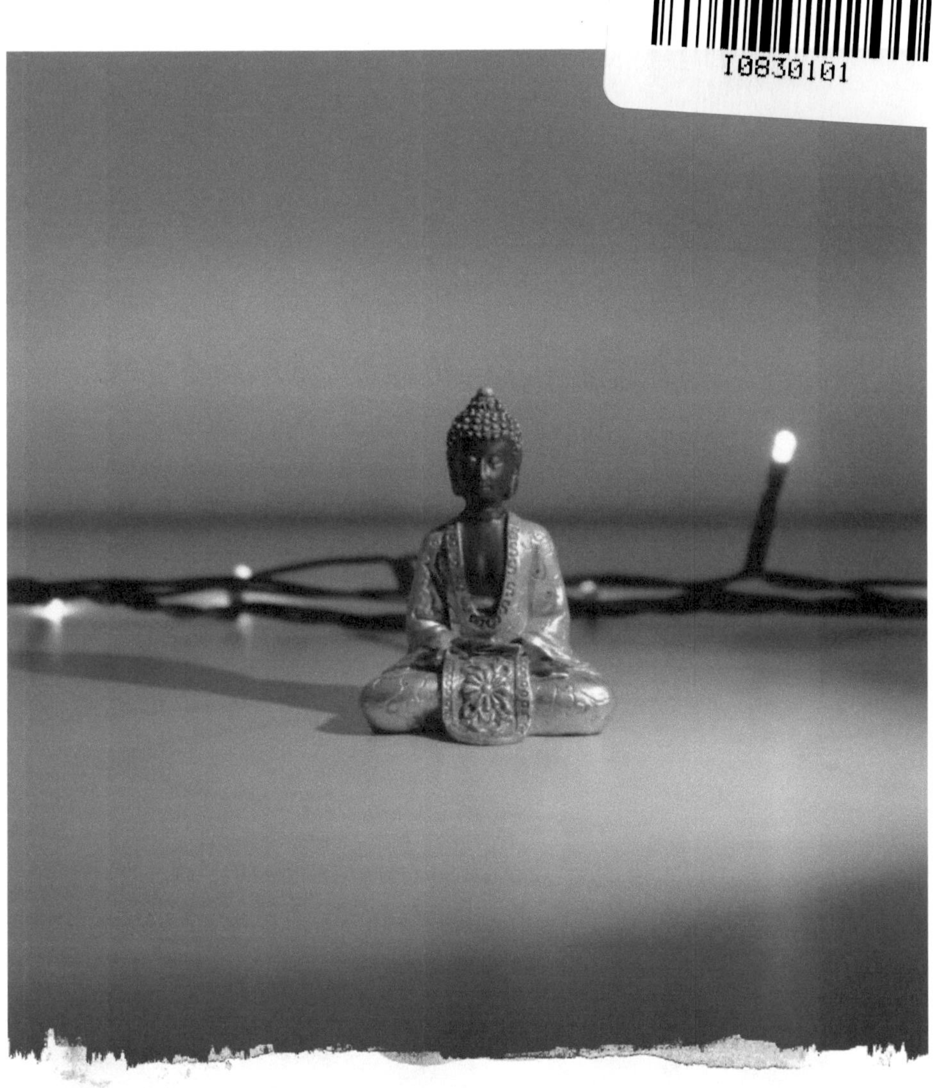

"Happiness lies **in us**, not in things." – Buddah

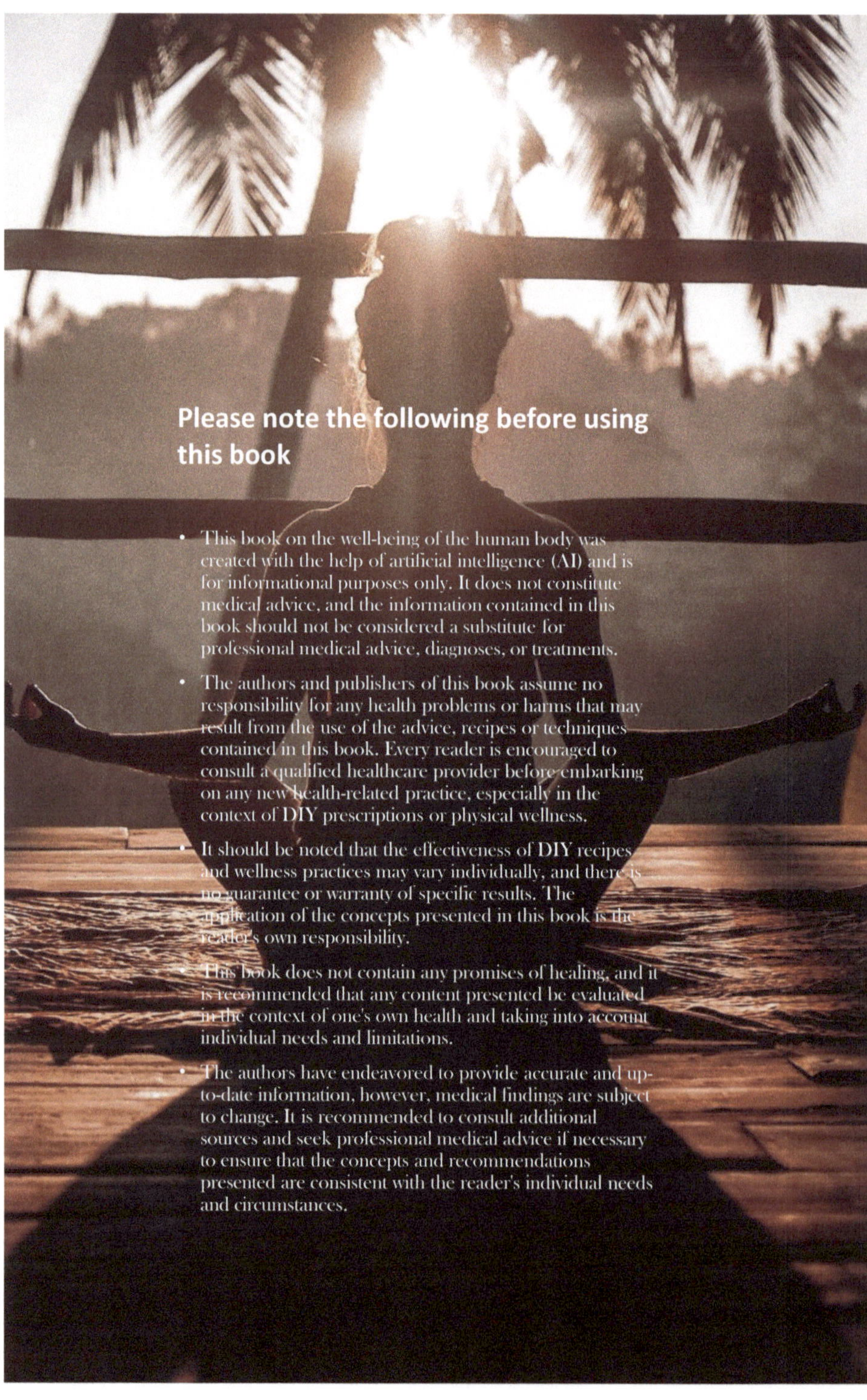

Please note the following before using this book

- This book on the well-being of the human body was created with the help of artificial intelligence (AI) and is for informational purposes only. It does not constitute medical advice, and the information contained in this book should not be considered a substitute for professional medical advice, diagnoses, or treatments.

- The authors and publishers of this book assume no responsibility for any health problems or harms that may result from the use of the advice, recipes or techniques contained in this book. Every reader is encouraged to consult a qualified healthcare provider before embarking on any new health-related practice, especially in the context of DIY prescriptions or physical wellness.

- It should be noted that the effectiveness of DIY recipes and wellness practices may vary individually, and there is no guarantee or warranty of specific results. The application of the concepts presented in this book is the reader's own responsibility.

- This book does not contain any promises of healing, and it is recommended that any content presented be evaluated in the context of one's own health and taking into account individual needs and limitations.

- The authors have endeavored to provide accurate and up-to-date information, however, medical findings are subject to change. It is recommended to consult additional sources and seek professional medical advice if necessary to ensure that the concepts and recommendations presented are consistent with the reader's individual needs and circumstances.

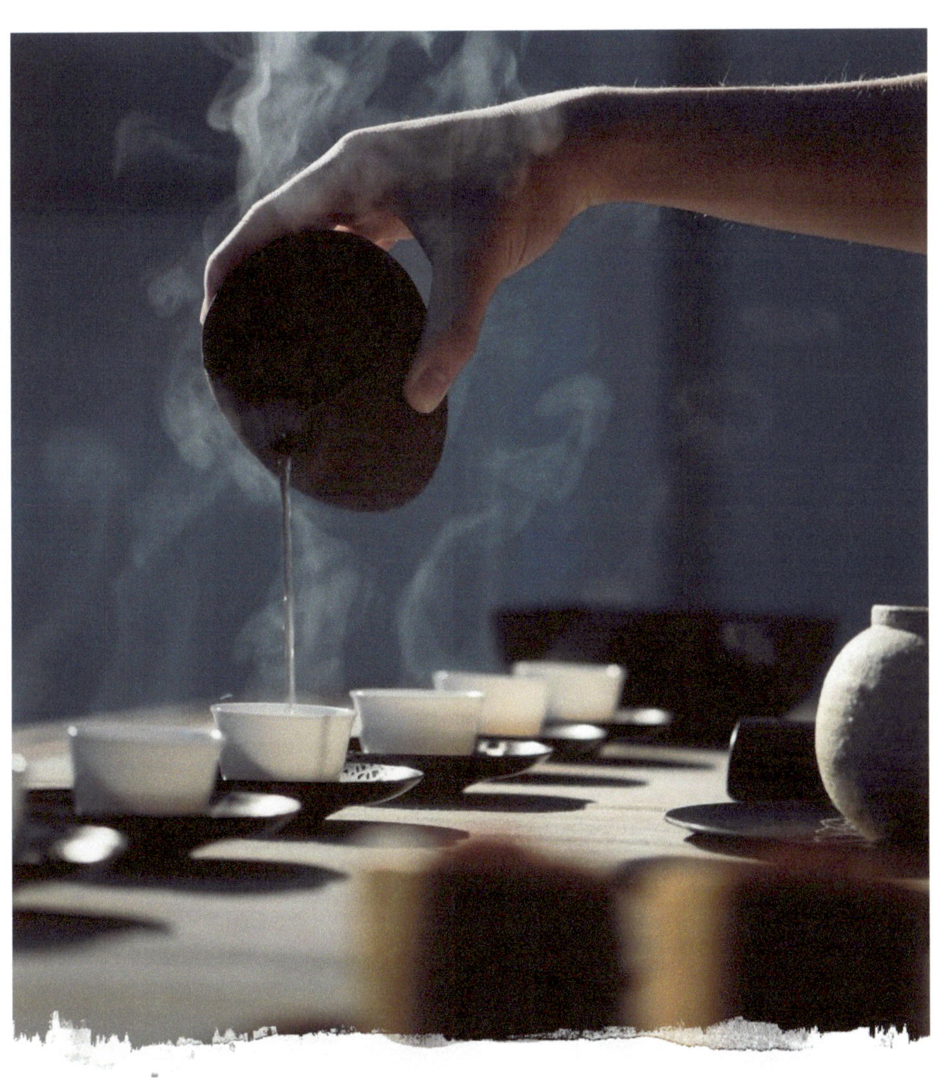

Recipes for the body

Honey Cinnamon Blend for Sore Throat:
Ingredients: 1 tsp honey, 1/2 tsp cinnamon
How to use: Take mixture to relieve sore throat.

Garlic Oil for Earache:
Ingredients: 3 cloves of garlic, 2 tbsp olive oil
Application: Heat garlic in oil, let cool, drip into the painful ear.

Chamomile tea for stomach discomfort:
Ingredients: 1 chamomile tea bag, 1 cup hot water
Application: Prepare tea, drink slowly to soothe stomach discomfort.

Garlic Honey Syrup for Cough:
Ingredients: Minced garlic (2 cloves of garlic), honey (2 tablespoons)
Effect: Relieves coughs and strengthens the immune system.

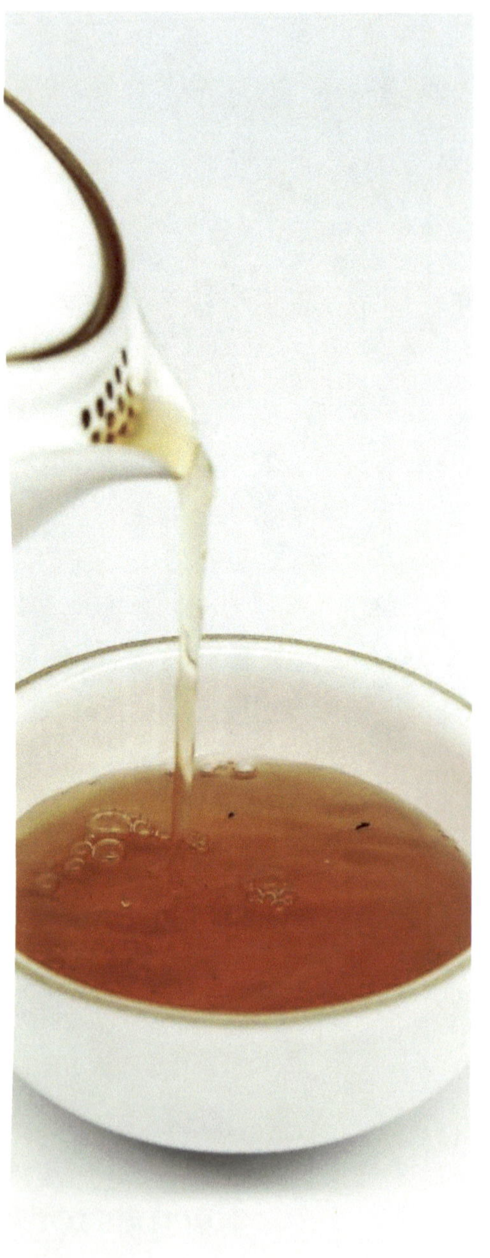

Apple cider vinegar for heartburn:
Ingredients: 1 tbsp apple cider vinegar, 1 glass of water
How to use: Mix vinegar in water, drink before meals to reduce heartburn.

Saltwater Gargling for Sore Throat:
Ingredients: 1 tsp salt, 1 glass of warm water
How to use: Gargle with the solution to relieve a sore throat.

Eucalyptus vapor for nasal congestion:
Ingredients: A few drops of eucalyptus oil, hot water
Application: Add eucalyptus oil to the hot water, inhale to open the airways.

Turmeric Milk Against Inflammation:
Ingredients: 1 tsp turmeric powder, 1 cup milk, honey to taste
Application: Dissolve turmeric in warm milk, sweeten with honey, drink before bedtime.

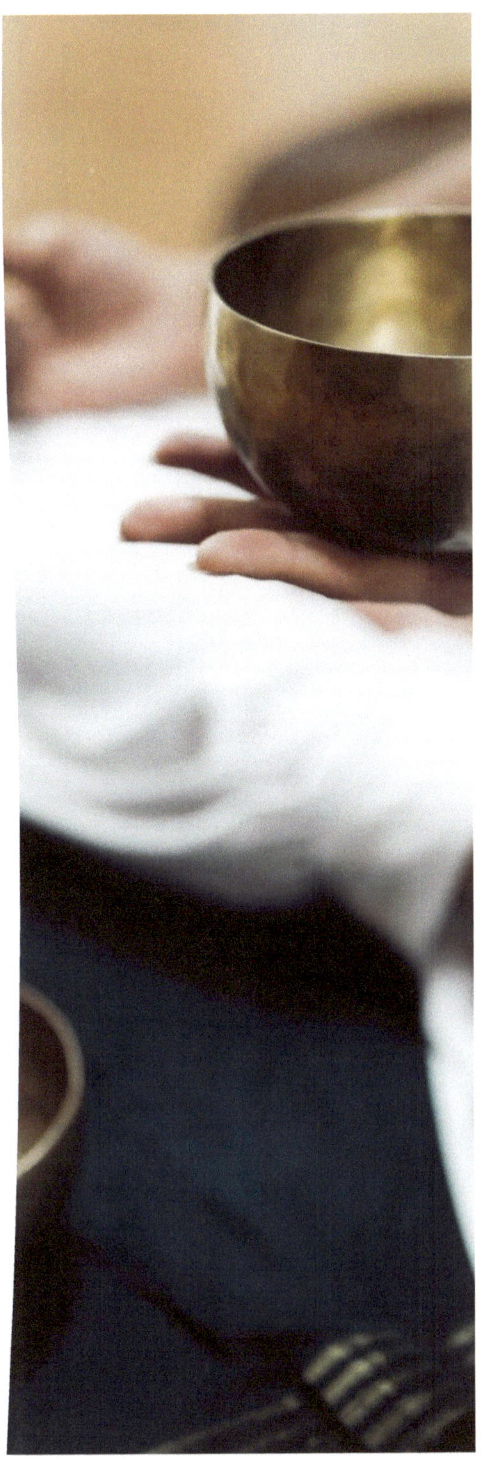

**Aloe Vera Gel for
Sunburn:**
Ingredients: Fresh aloe vera gel
How to use: Apply gel to
sunburned skin.

**Rosemary oil for
headaches:**
Ingredients: A few drops of
rosemary oil, carrier oil (e.g.
almond oil)
Application: Mix oils, rub on
temples and forehead to relieve
headaches.

Peppermint oil for nausea:
Ingredients: A few drops of
peppermint oil, carrier oil
How to use: Apply diluted to
the wrists to relieve nausea.

**Pumpkin seeds for bladder
problems:**
Ingredients: Handful of
pumpkin seeds
How to use: Eat a handful of
pumpkin seeds daily to prevent
bladder problems.

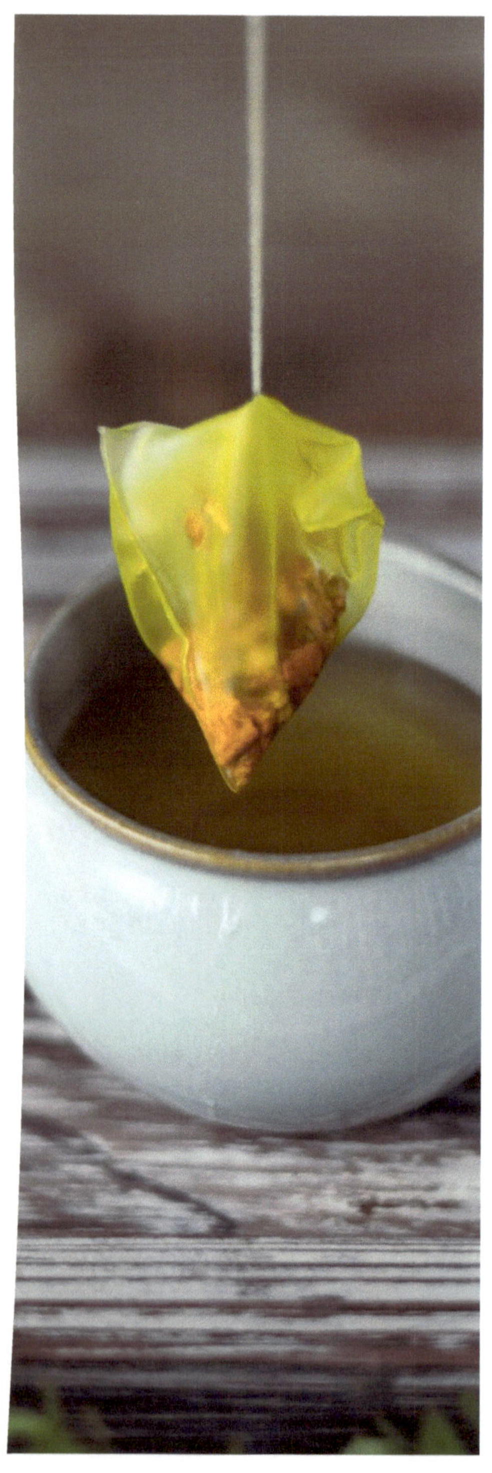

Lemon Honey Gargle Solution for Sore Throat:
Ingredients: lemon juice (1 tablespoon), honey (1 tablespoon), warm water
Effect: Reduces sore throat and has an anti-inflammatory effect.

Peppermint oil for headaches:
Ingredients: peppermint oil (a few drops), carrier oil (e.g. almond oil)
Effect: Relieves headaches and promotes relaxation.

Hot onion wraps for earaches:
Ingredients: peeled onion (1), cotton cloth
Effect: Relieves earache due to anti-inflammatory properties.

Rosemary oil for migraines:
Ingredients: rosemary oil (a few drops), carrier oil
Effect: Reduces migraine symptoms and promotes blood circulation.

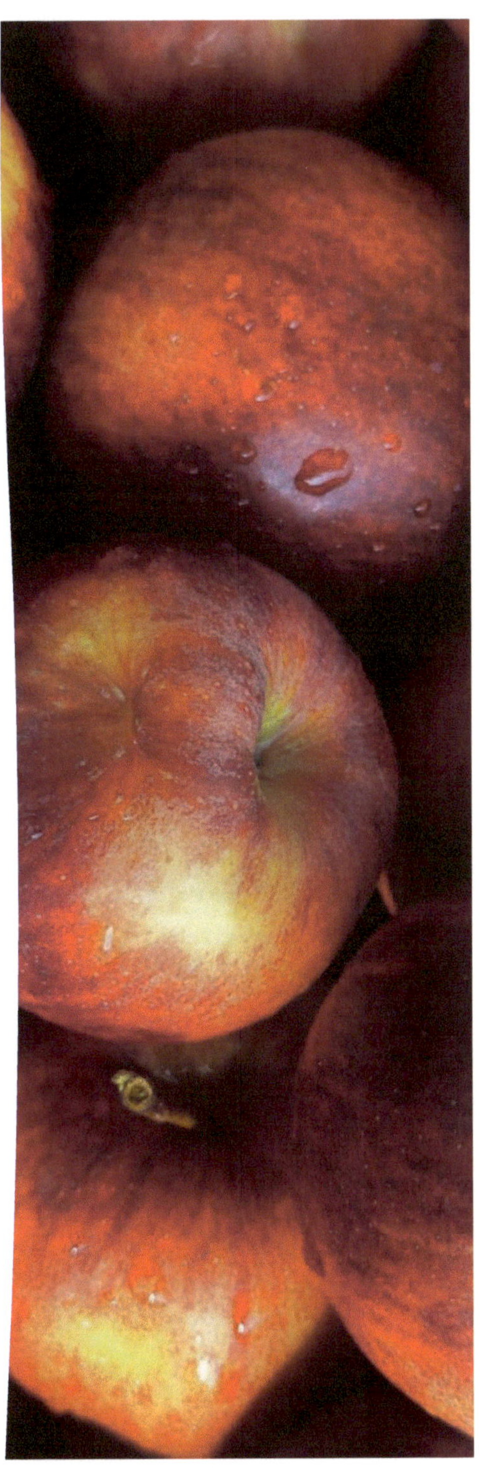

Aloe Vera Gel for Sunburn:
Ingredients: Fresh aloe vera gel (directly from the plant)
Effect: Cooling effect, relieves pain and promotes healing from sunburn.

Thyme tea for cough:
Ingredients: 1 tsp dried thyme, 1 cup hot water
How to use: Prepare tea, drink slowly to relieve cough.

Radish cough syrup:
Ingredients: 1 radish, 2 tbsp honey
Application: grate radish, add honey, extract juice, take for cough.

Chamomile steam bath for sinusitis:
Ingredients: Handful of chamomile flowers, hot water
Application: Add chamomile flowers to hot water, inhale steam to open blocked nasal passages.

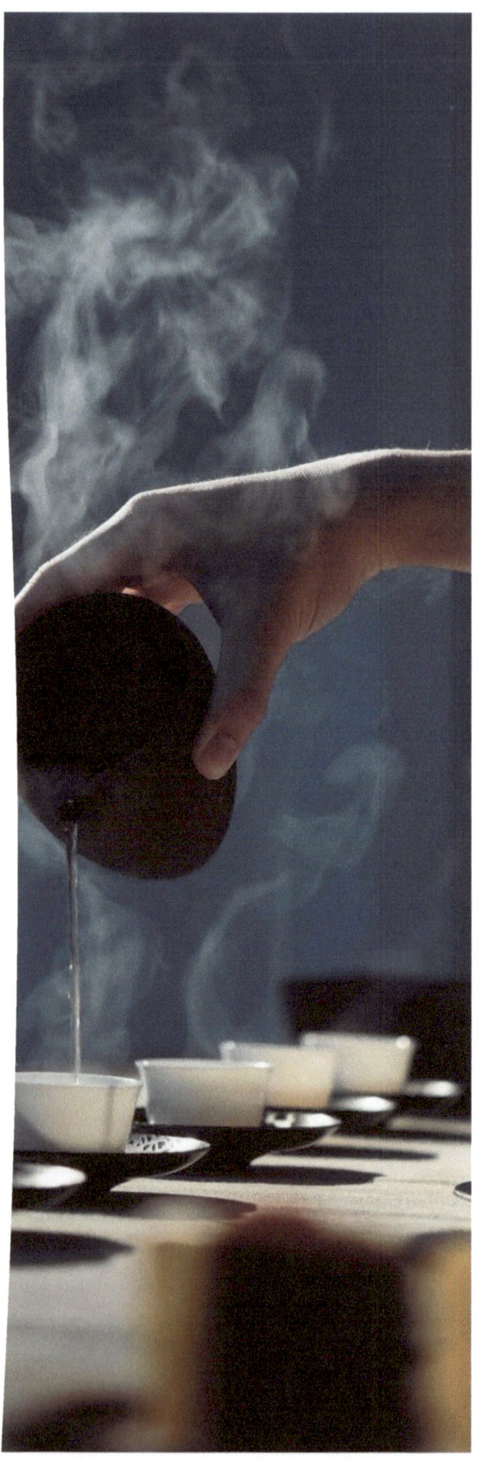

Cucumber Eye Mask for Puffiness:
Ingredients: Thin slices of cucumber
How to use: Place discs on closed eyes to reduce puffiness.

Mustard wrap for muscle pain:
Ingredients: 2 tbsp mustard powder, water as needed
Application: Make paste, apply to aching muscles, leave on for 15 minutes, wash off.

Oregano oil for skin infections:
Ingredients: A few drops of oregano oil, carrier oil (e.g. olive oil)
Application: Mix oils, apply to infected areas of the skin.

Thyme Honey Tea for Sore Throat:
Ingredients: 1 tsp dried thyme, 1 tbsp honey, 1 cup hot water
Application: Pour hot water over thyme, add honey, drink tea to relieve sore throat.

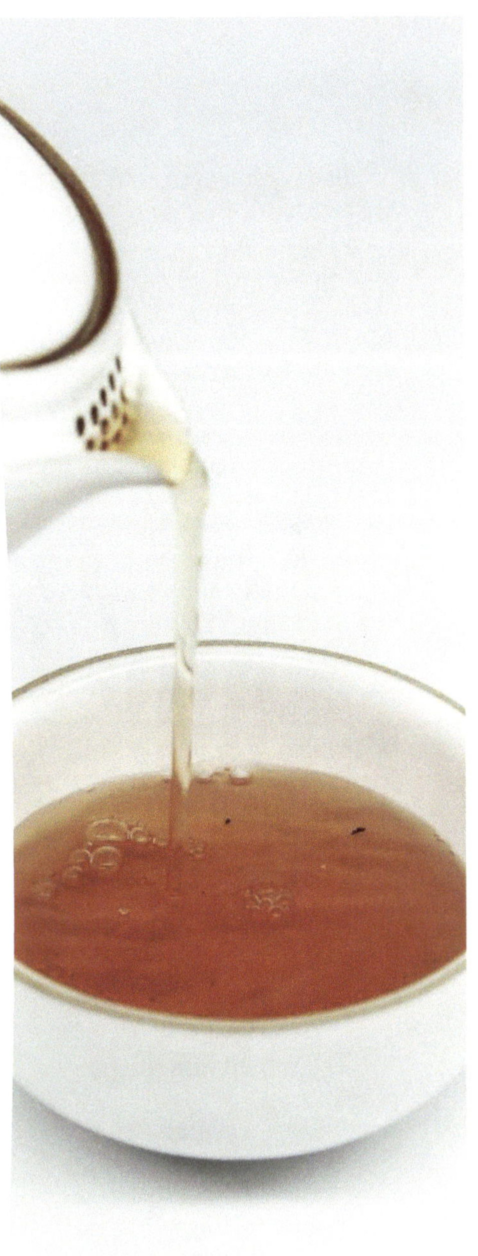

Mint-Lemon-Ginger Water for Detox:
Ingredients: A few mint leaves, juice of one lemon, 1 tsp grated ginger, 1 cup of warm water
Application: Mix ingredients, drink to detoxify the body.

Beetroot Cucumber Juice for Liver Cleanse:
Ingredients: 1 beetroot, 1/2 cucumber, 1 apple
Application: Juicing vegetables and fruits, drinking juice to support the liver.

Tomato & Honey Mask for Sunburn:
Ingredients: 1 ripe tomato, 1 tbsp honey
Application: Puree the tomato, mix with honey, apply to sunburned skin, leave on for 15 minutes, rinse.

Clove mouthwash for gum problems:
Ingredients: A few cloves, 1 cup of warm water
How to use: Add cloves to warm water, use as a mouthwash to alleviate gum problems.

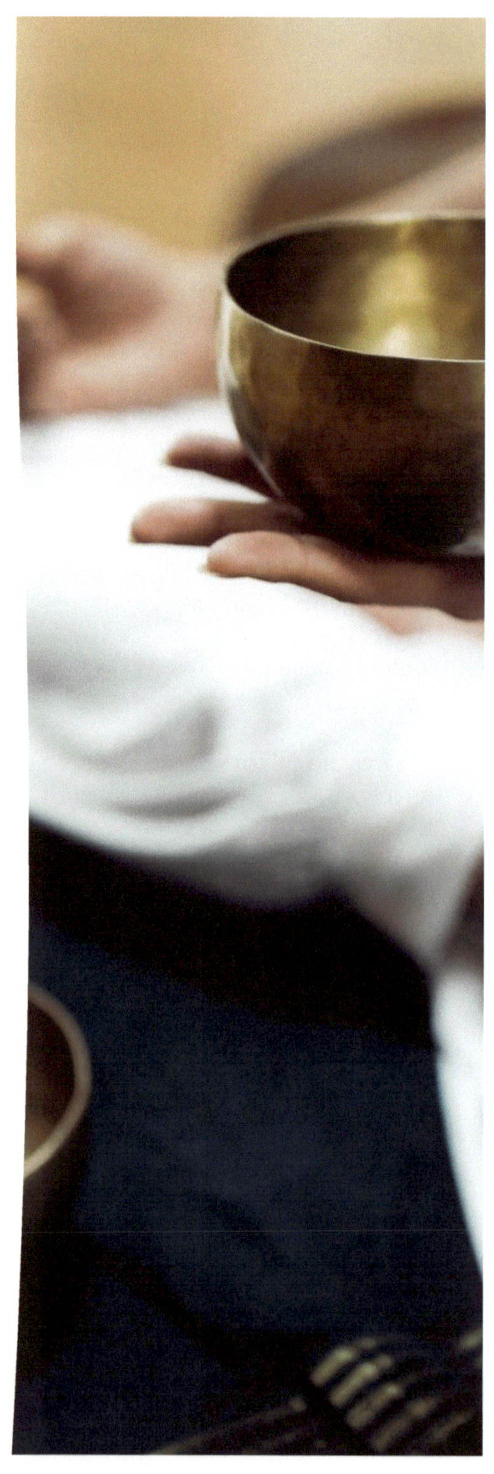

**Curd Mint Face Mask for
Pimples:**
Ingredients: 2 tbsp quark, a few
fresh mint leaves
How to use: Mix ingredients, apply
to the face, leave on for 15
minutes, rinse.

**Ginger Tea with Lemon for
Cold:**
Ingredients: 1 tsp fresh grated
ginger, juice of one lemon, 1 tbsp
honey, 1 cup of hot water
Application: Pour hot water over
ginger, add lemon and honey,
drink tea to relieve cold symptoms.

**Onion cough syrup against
cough irritation:**
Ingredients: 1 chopped onion, 2
tbsp honey
Application: Mix onion with honey,
leave to infuse overnight, take
syrup for cough.

**Marjoram Potato Wrap for
Headaches:**
Ingredients: A few sprigs of
marjoram, boiled potatoes
Application: Mix sprigs of
marjoram with boiled potatoes,
place on the forehead to relieve
headaches.

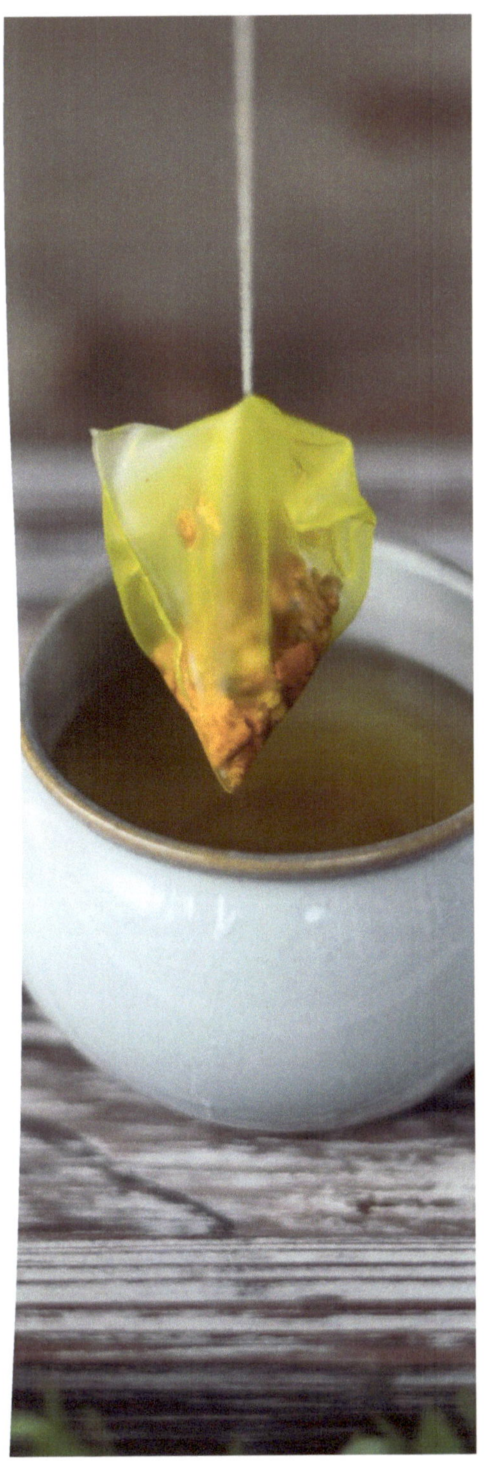

Sage Chamomile Gargle Solution for Sore Throat:
Ingredients: 1 tsp dried sage leaves, 1 tsp dried chamomile flowers, 1 cup warm water
Application: Pour warm water over herbs, strain, use as gargle solution.

Eucalyptus Steam Inhalation for Respiratory Problems:
Ingredients: A few drops of eucalyptus oil, hot water
Application: Add oil to hot water, inhale steam to relieve respiratory symptoms.

St. John's wort oil for minor burns:
Ingredients: Dried St. John's wort flowers, olive oil
Application: Pickle flowers in oil, store in a sunny place, apply oil to minor burns.

Banana peels for warts:
Ingredients: Inside of a banana peel
Application: Place banana peel on the wart, fix with a bandage, leave on overnight.

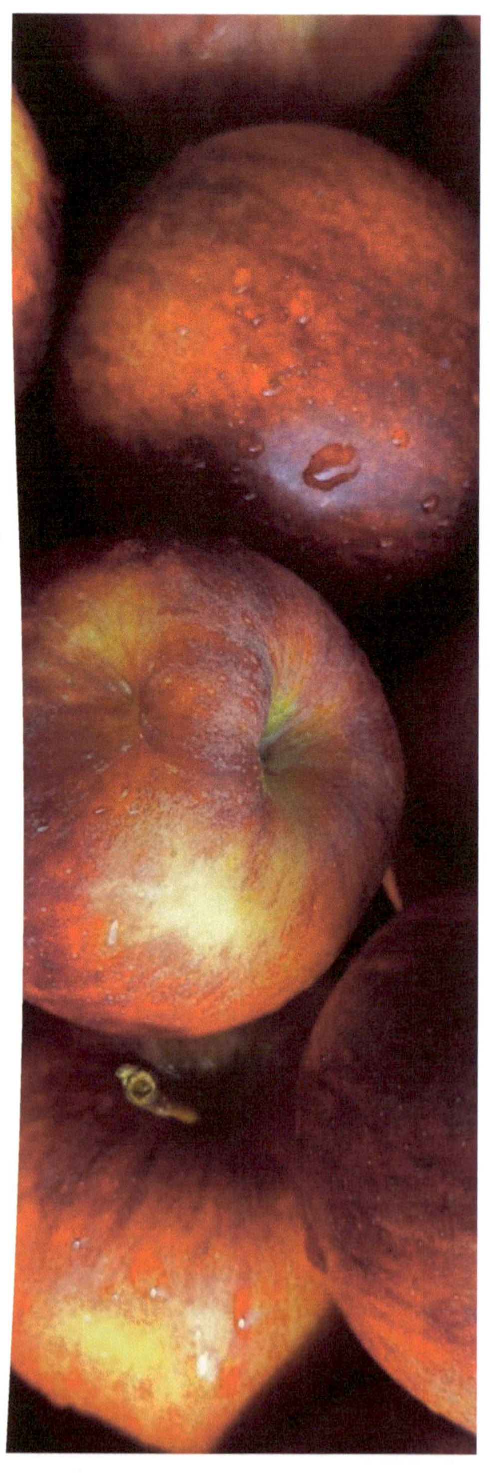

Parsley for bad breath:
Ingredients: Handful of fresh
parsley
How to use: Chew parsley to
combat bad breath.

**Sage tea for inflammation in
the mouth area:**
Ingredients: 1 tsp dried sage
leaves, 1 cup hot water
Application: Prepare tea, let it
cool, use as a mouthwash.

**Fennel Honey Tea for
Stomach Cramps:**
Ingredients: 1 tsp fennel seeds,
1 tbsp honey, 1 cup hot water
Application: Pour hot water
over fennel seeds, add honey,
drink to relieve stomach
cramps.

**Celery smoothie for water
retention:**
Ingredients: 1 celery stalk, 1
green apple, 1 cup water
How to use: Mix ingredients,
drink daily to reduce water
retention.

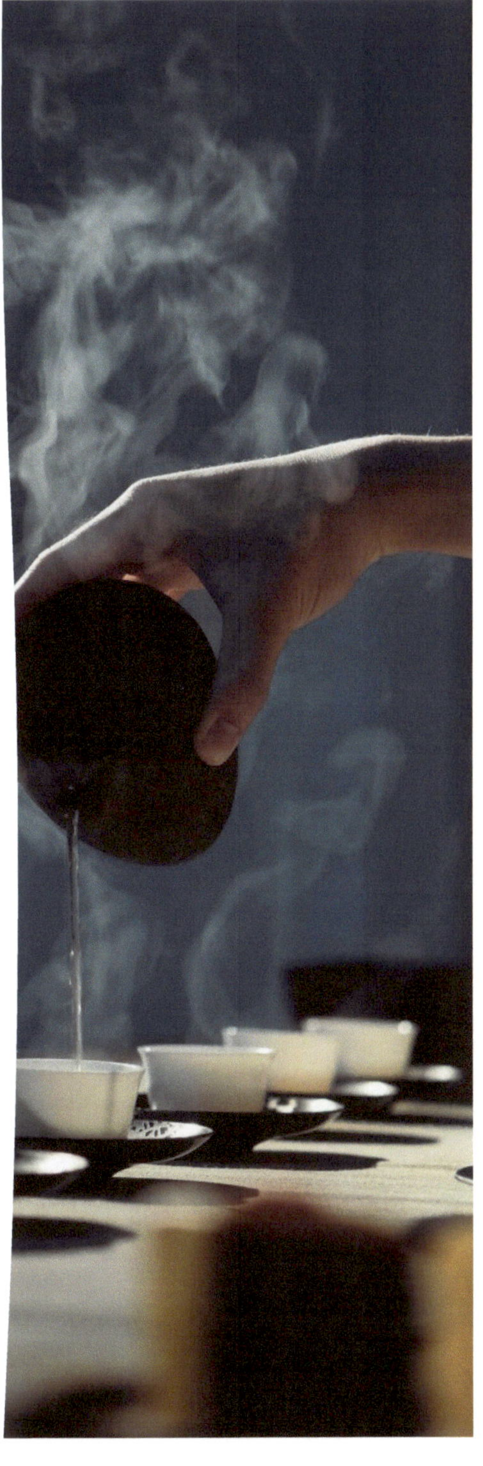

Menthol steam inhalation for respiratory problems:
Ingredients: A few drops of menthol oil, hot water
Application: Add menthol oil to hot water, inhale steam to relieve respiratory discomfort.

Tomato Face Scrub for Blackheads:
Ingredients: 1 ripe tomato, 1 tsp sugar
How to use: Puree the tomato, add sugar, apply as a scrub, leave on for 10 minutes, rinse.

Elderberry syrup for cold:
Ingredients: Handful of elderberries, 1 cup water, 2 tbsp honey
Application: boil berries, strain, add honey, take syrup for cold.

Arugula & Cucumber Smoothie for Digestion:
Ingredients: A handful of arugula, 1/2 cucumber, 1 cup water
Application: Mix ingredients, drink as a smoothie to promote digestion.

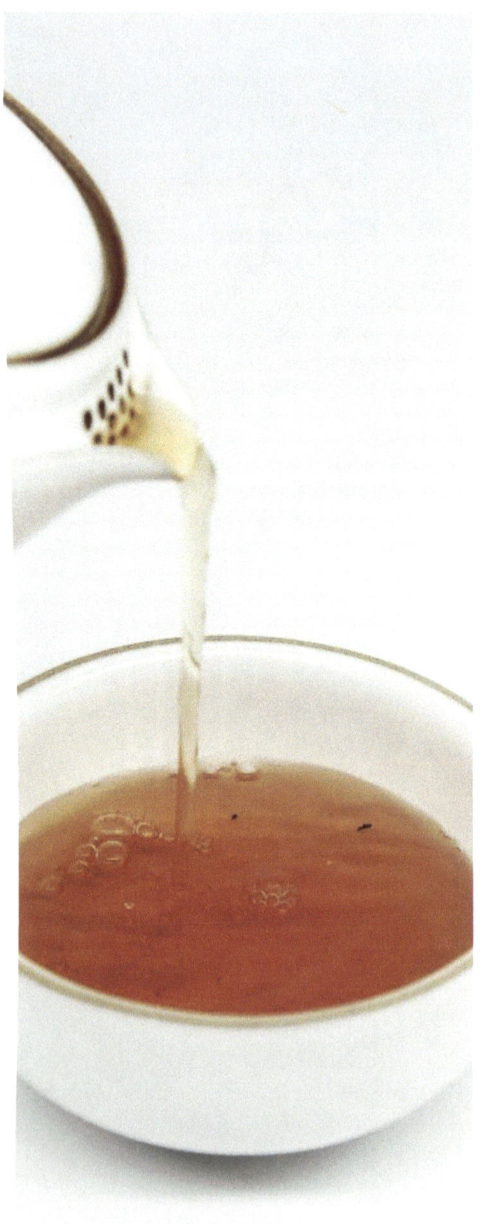

Potato slices for dark circles:
Ingredients: Thin potato slices
How to use: Place discs on closed eyes to reduce dark circles.

Nettle tea for allergic reactions:
Ingredients: 1 tsp dried nettle leaves, 1 cup hot water
Application: Pour hot water over leaves, strain, drink tea to alleviate allergic reactions.

Peppermint tea for breath freshness:
Ingredients: 1 tsp dried peppermint leaves, 1 cup hot water
Application: Pour hot water over the leaves, strain, drink as a tea to promote breathlessness.

Chamomile oil for skin irritations:
Ingredients: 2 tsp dried chamomile flowers, almond oil
Application: Soak flowers in oil, strain, apply oil to irritated areas of skin.

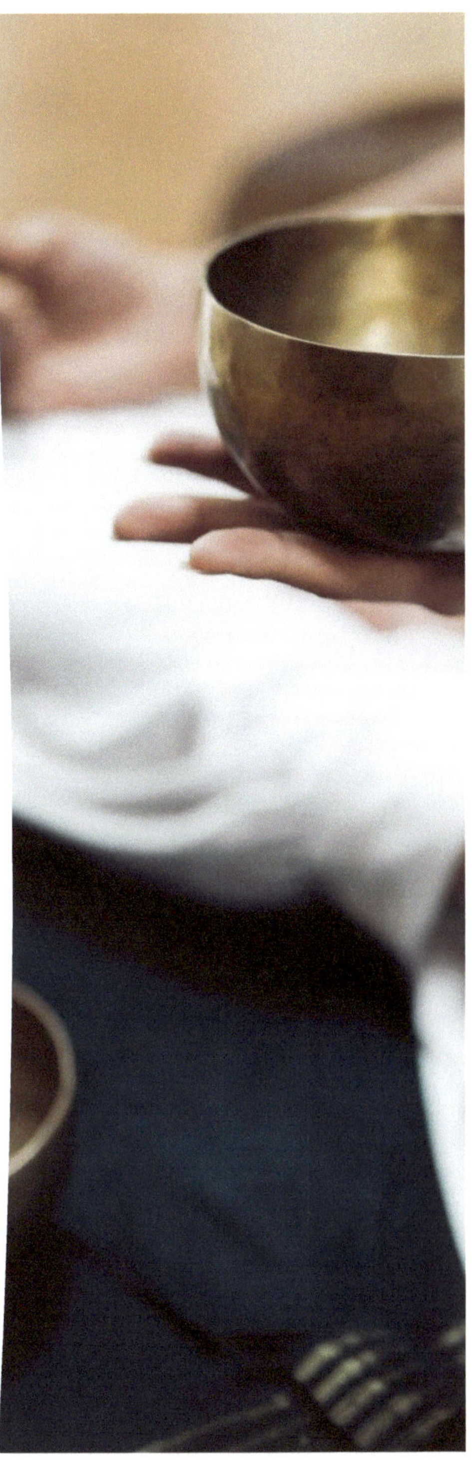

Blackcurrant juice for joint pain:
Ingredients: Handful of fresh blackcurrants, water as needed
Application: boil berries, strain, drink juice to relieve joint pain.

Aloe Vera Cucumber Facial Spray for Skin Irritation:
Ingredients: 2 tbsp aloe vera gel, 1/4 cup cucumber juice
Application: Pour mixture into a spray bottle, spray on the face to soothe skin irritation.

Turmeric Face Mask for Acne:
Ingredients: 1 tsp turmeric powder, 1 tbsp plain yoghurt
How to use: Apply mixture to face, leave on for 15 minutes, rinse.

Potato juice for stomach problems:
Ingredients: 1 large potato
Application: Juicing potato, drinking juice to relieve stomach problems.

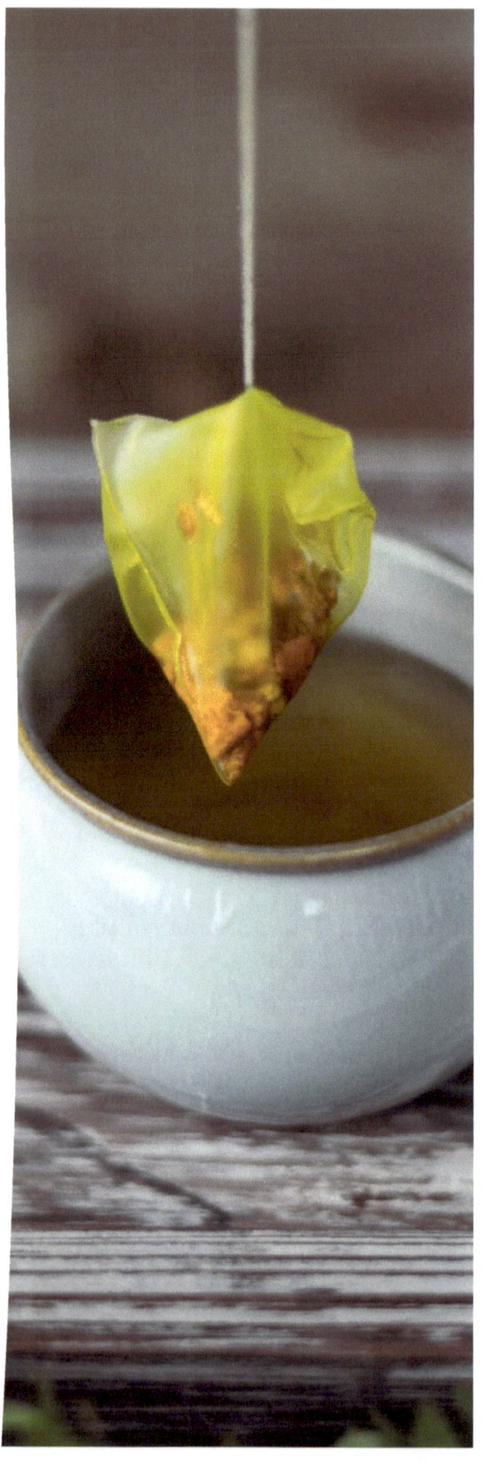

Orange Oil Aromatherapy for Headaches:
Ingredients: A few drops of orange oil, diffuser
How to use: Add oil to the diffuser to relieve headaches.

Sage Honey Gargle Solution for Sore Throat:
Ingredients: 1 tsp dried sage leaves, 1 tsp honey, 1 cup warm water
How to use: Gargle mixture to relieve sore throat.

Chia Seed Tea for Digestion:
Ingredients: 1 tbsp chia seeds, 1 cup hot water
How to use: Add chia seeds to hot water, let them swell, drink them to promote digestion.

Ginger Lemon Tea for Nausea:
Ingredients: 1 tsp fresh grated ginger, juice of half a lemon, 1 cup of hot water
How to use: Add ginger and lemon juice to hot water, drink to relieve nausea.

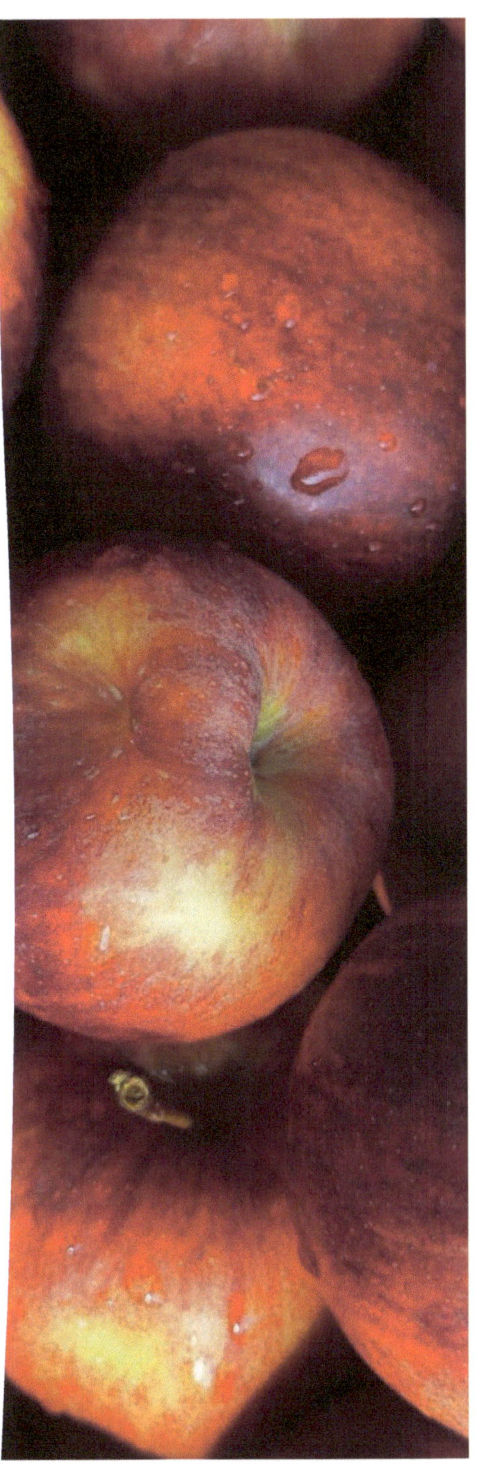

Beetroot Juice for Liver Health:
Ingredients: 1 beetroot, 1 apple
Application: Juice beets and apple, drink juice to promote liver health.

Lemon Garlic Cough Syrup:
Ingredients: juice of one lemon, 2 cloves of garlic, 1 tbsp honey
Application: Mix lemon juice with crushed garlic and honey, take against cough.

Honey Onion Cough Syrup:
Ingredients: 1 chopped onion, 2 tbsp honey
Application: Mix onion with honey, leave to infuse overnight, take syrup for cough.

Eucalyptus Thyme Steam Inhalation for Respiratory Problems:
Ingredients: A few drops of eucalyptus oil, a few sprigs of thyme, hot water
Application: Add oil and thyme to hot water, inhale steam to relieve breathing problems.

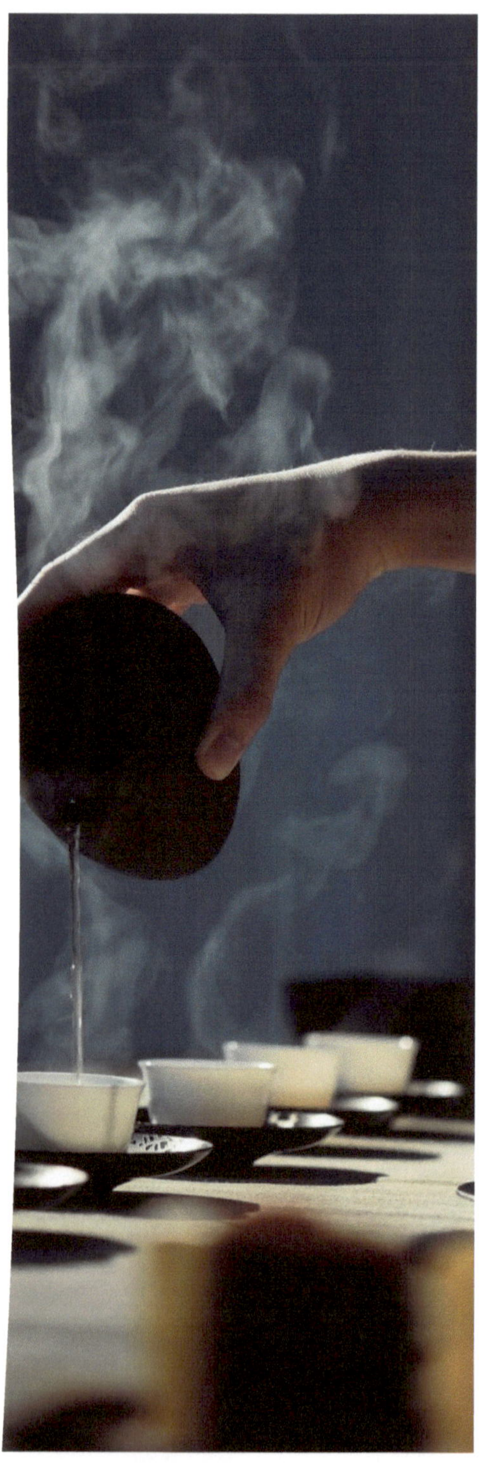

Parsley tea for flatulence:
Ingredients: A handful of fresh parsley, 1 cup of hot water
How to use: Pour hot water over parsley, strain, drink tea to reduce flatulence.

Garlic Honey Mask for Pimples:
Ingredients: 2 cloves of garlic, 1 tbsp honey
Application: Press garlic, mix with honey, apply as a mask to pimples, leave on for 10 minutes, rinse.

Chamomile Tea Ice Cubes for Puffy Eyes:
Ingredients: chamomile tea, ice cube tray
How to use: Freeze chamomile tea, gently use ice cubes under the eyes to reduce puffiness.

Chamomile Honey Eye Compress for Redness:
Ingredients: chamomile tea, 1 tbsp honey
Application: boil tea, let it cool, add honey, soak cotton pads, put on closed eyes to relieve redness.

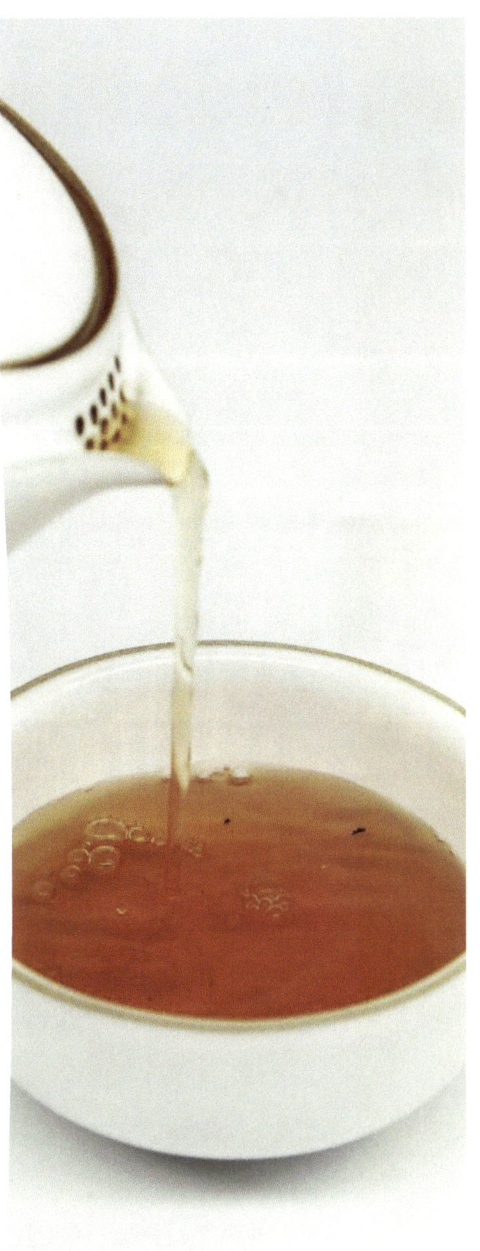

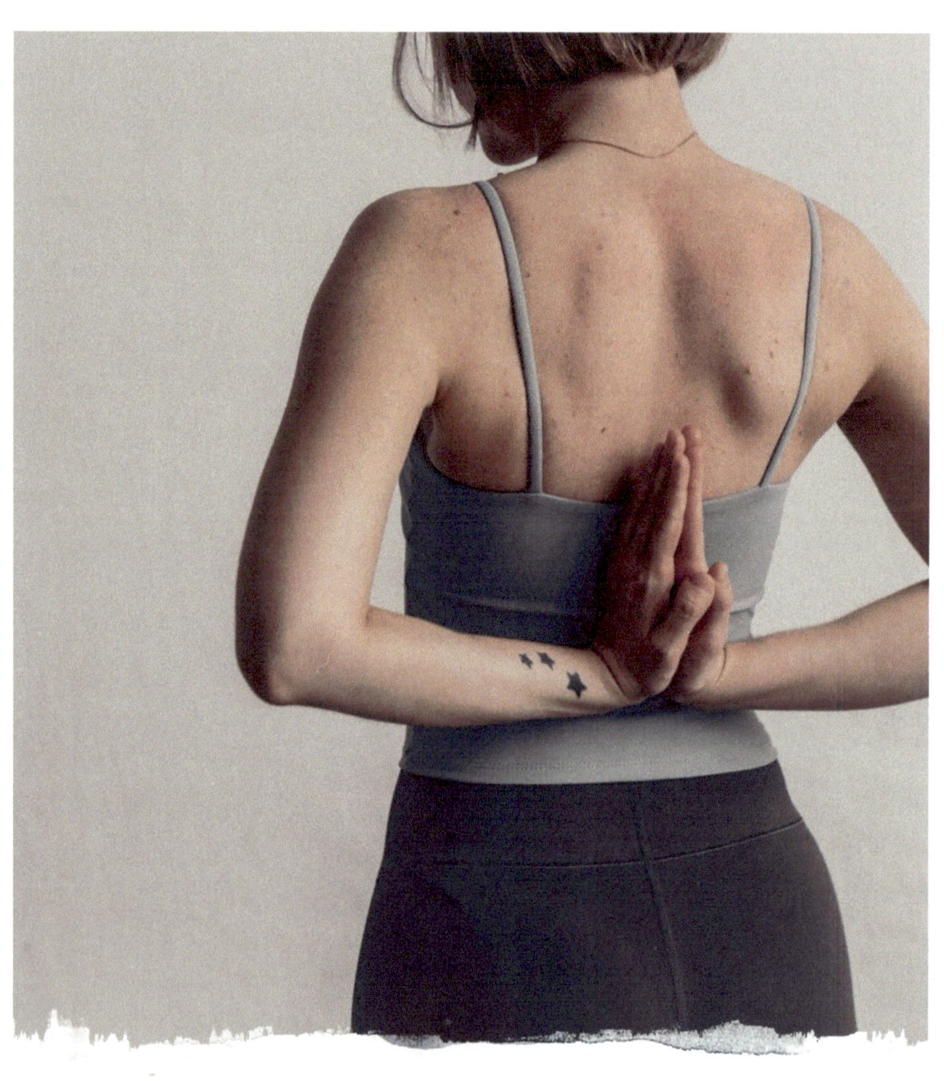

Recipes for the soul

Coconut Oil for Skin Care:
Ingredients: Natural coconut oil
How to use: Use as a moisturizer
for the skin.

Yogurt mask for skin:
 Ingredients: Natural yoghurt,
honey
How to use: Apply mixture to
face, leave on for 15 minutes,
rinse.

Apple cider vinegar for skin:
 Ingredients: apple cider vinegar
(1 part), water (1 part)
Effect: Improves the appearance
of the skin and is effective against
acne.

**Oatmeal bath for sensitive
skin:**
Ingredients: rolled oats (1 cup),
warm bath water
Effect: Soothes the skin and
relieves itching.

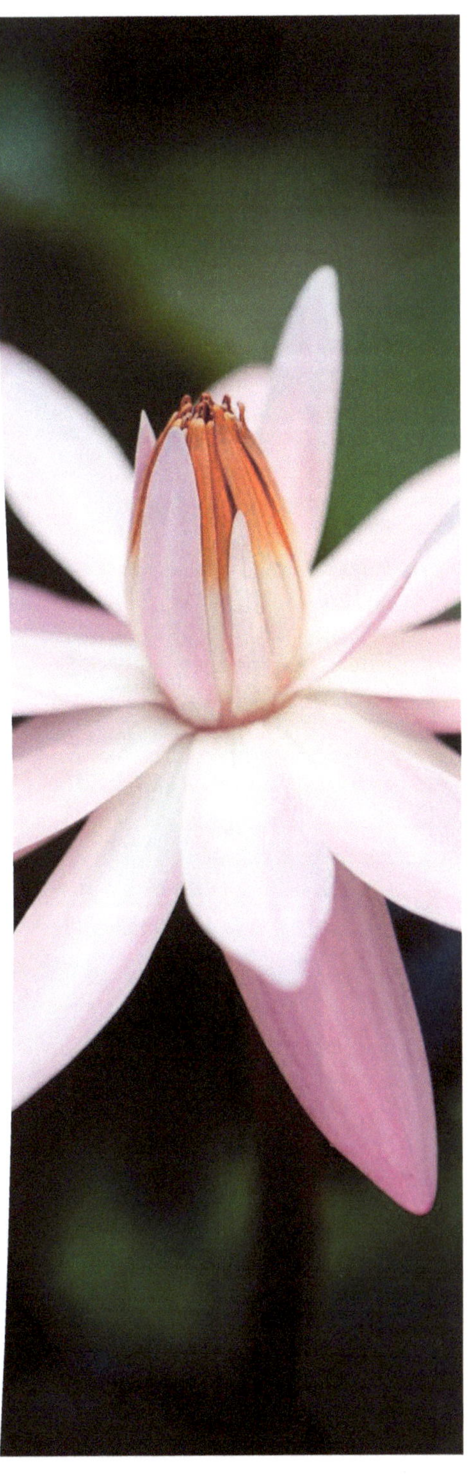

Coconut Oil Toothpaste for Whiter Teeth:
Ingredients: coconut oil (2 tablespoons), baking soda (1 tablespoon)
Effect: Natural teeth whitening and gum care.

Yogurt Honey Mask for Skin:
Ingredients: natural yogurt (2 tablespoons), honey (1 tablespoon)
Effect: Hydrates the skin and reduces blemishes.

Lavender oil for better sleep:
Ingredients: lavender oil (a few drops), aroma lamp or cloth
Effect: Promotes relaxation and improves sleep.

Oatmeal Honey Face Mask:
Ingredients: 2 tbsp rolled oats, 1 tbsp honey, water as needed
How to use: Mix into a paste, apply to the face, leave on for 15 minutes, rinse.

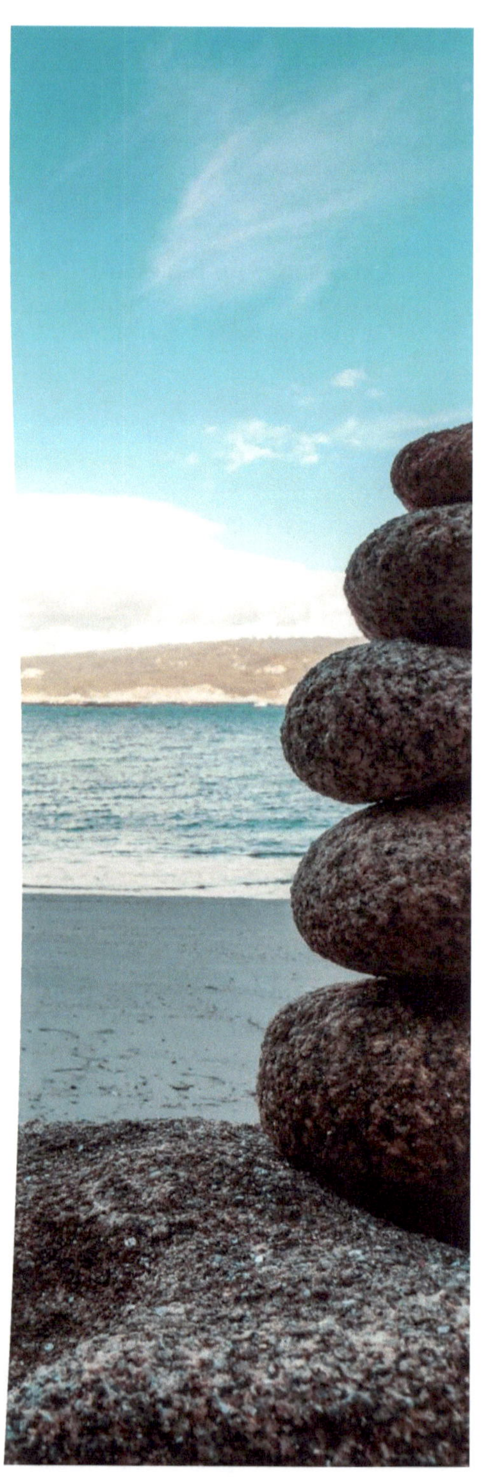

Turmeric Toothpaste for Whiter Teeth:
Ingredients: 1 tsp turmeric powder, 1 tsp coconut oil
Application: Mix into a paste, apply to teeth, leave on for 5 minutes, rinse thoroughly.

Blueberry Honey Tea for Eye Health:
Ingredients: Handful of blueberries, 1 tbsp honey
Application: Brew berries in hot water, strain, add honey, drink for eye health.

Apple Cider Vinegar for Digestion:
Ingredients: 1 tbsp apple cider vinegar, 1 glass of water
How to use: Dissolve vinegar in water, drink before meals to aid digestion.

Rosewater Facial Toner:
Ingredients: 2 tbsp rose water
How to use: Transfer to a cotton pad, use facial toner to refresh the skin.

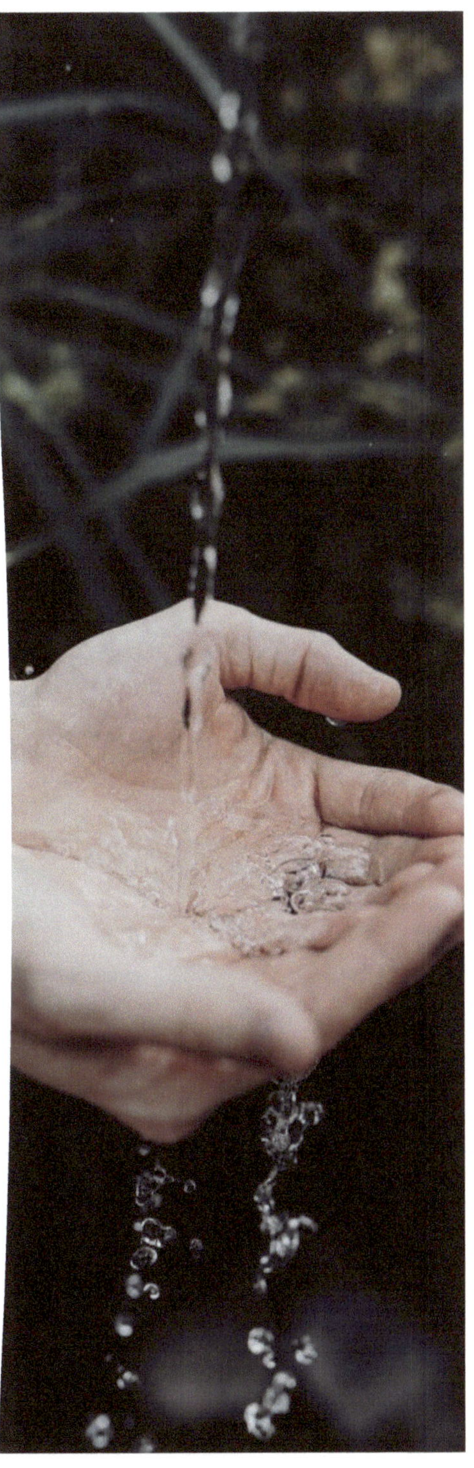

Coconut Oil Lemon Hair Treatment:
Ingredients: 2 tbsp coconut oil, juice of half a lemon
How to use: Apply mixture to hair, leave on for 30 minutes, rinse.

Chamomilla globules for insomnia:
Ingredients: Chamomilla globules (according to package instructions)
How to use: Take globules before bedtime to relieve insomnia.

Avocado Honey Face Mask for Dry Skin:
Ingredients: 1/2 ripe avocado, 1 tbsp honey
How to use: Puree the avocado, mix with honey, apply to the face, leave on for 15 minutes, rinse.

Coconut Oil Lemon Scrub for Lips:
Ingredients: 1 tsp coconut oil, 1 tsp sugar, juice of half a lemon
Application: Mix ingredients, apply to lips, massage gently, rinse.

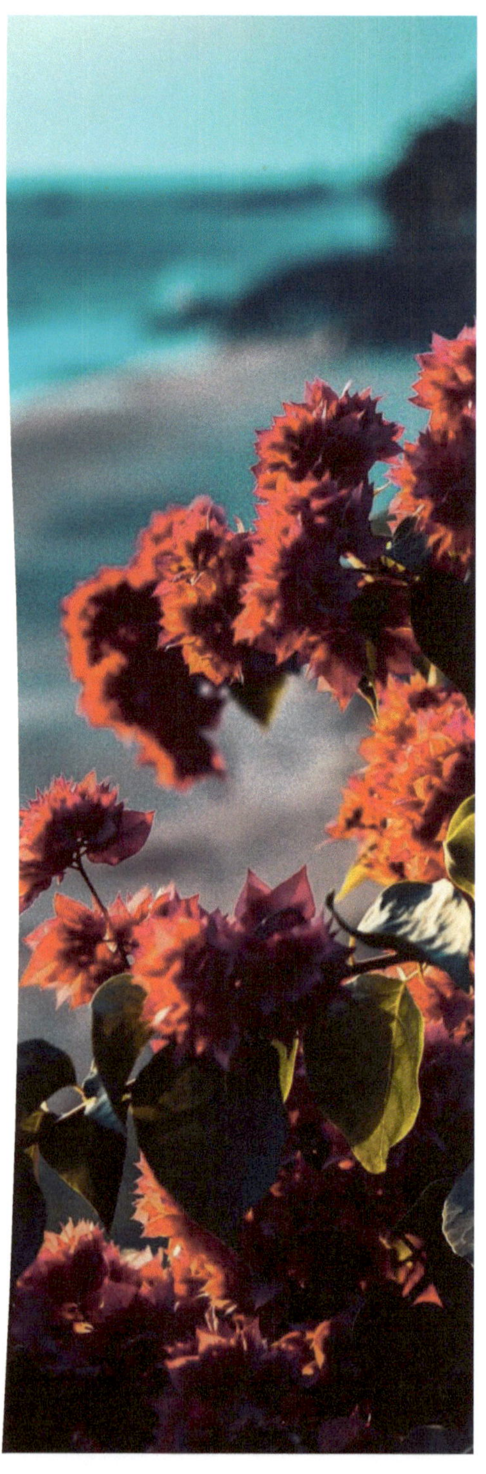

Apple Cider Vinegar Hair Conditioner for Shine:
Ingredients: 2 tbsp apple cider vinegar, 1 cup water
How to use: After shampooing, use as a final conditioner to add shine to the hair.

Pumpkin Honey Mask for Glowing Skin:
Ingredients: 2 tbsp pumpkin puree, 1 tbsp honey
How to use: Apply mixture to the face, leave on for 20 minutes, rinse.

Papaya Hair Mask for Volume:
Ingredients: 1/2 ripe papaya, 1 tbsp yoghurt
How to use: Puree papaya, mix with yoghurt, apply to hair, leave on for 30 minutes, rinse.

Basil Honey Tea for Stress Relief:
Ingredients: Handful of fresh basil leaves, 1 tbsp honey
Application: Brew basil leaves with hot water, add honey, drink to relieve stress.

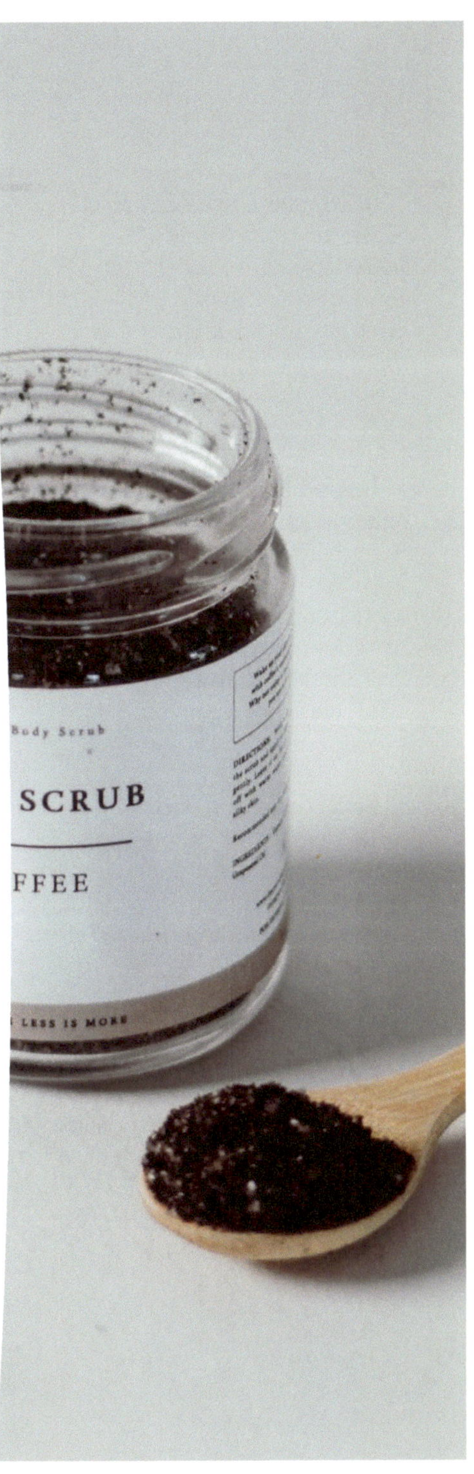

**Rosewater Cucumber Eye
Mask for Dark Circles:**
Ingredients: rose water, thin
slices of cucumber
How to use: Soak cucumber
slices in rose water, place on the
eyes to reduce dark circles.

**Lemon balm valerian tea for
better sleep:**
Ingredients: 1 tsp dried lemon
balm leaves, 1 tsp dried valerian
root, 1 cup hot water
Application: Pour hot water
over the leaves and roots, strain,
drink tea before going to bed.

**Potato juice for skin
lightening:**
Ingredients: 1 large potato
How to use: Juicing the potato,
applying juice to the skin to
lighten dark spots.

**Oatmeal Honey Face Mask
for Sensitive Skin:**
Ingredients: 2 tbsp rolled oats, 1
tbsp honey, water as needed
How to use: Mix oatmeal with
honey, apply to the face, leave
on for 15 minutes, rinse.

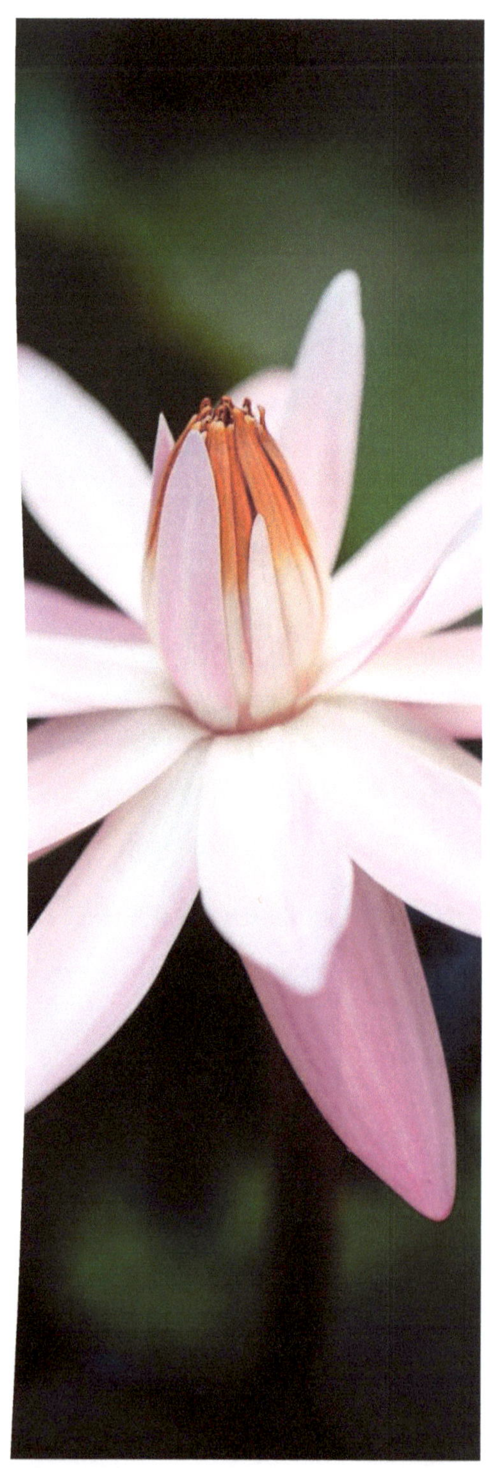

Salt Lemon Facial Scrub for Skin Renewal:
Ingredients: 1 tbsp sea salt, juice of half a lemon
How to use: Mix ingredients, apply to the face, massage gently, rinse.

Oatmeal Banana Mask for Skin Soothing:
Ingredients: 2 tbsp rolled oats, 1 ripe banana
Application: Puree oatmeal with banana, apply to the face, leave on for 20 minutes, rinse.

Coconut Oil Cinnamon Hair Treatment for Dry Scalp:
Ingredients: 2 tbsp coconut oil, 1 tsp cinnamon
How to use: Mix ingredients, apply to scalp, leave on for 30 minutes, rinse.

Papaya Honey Mask for Glowing Skin:
Ingredients: 1/2 ripe papaya, 1 tbsp honey
How to use: Puree papaya, mix with honey, apply to the face, leave on for 15 minutes, rinse.

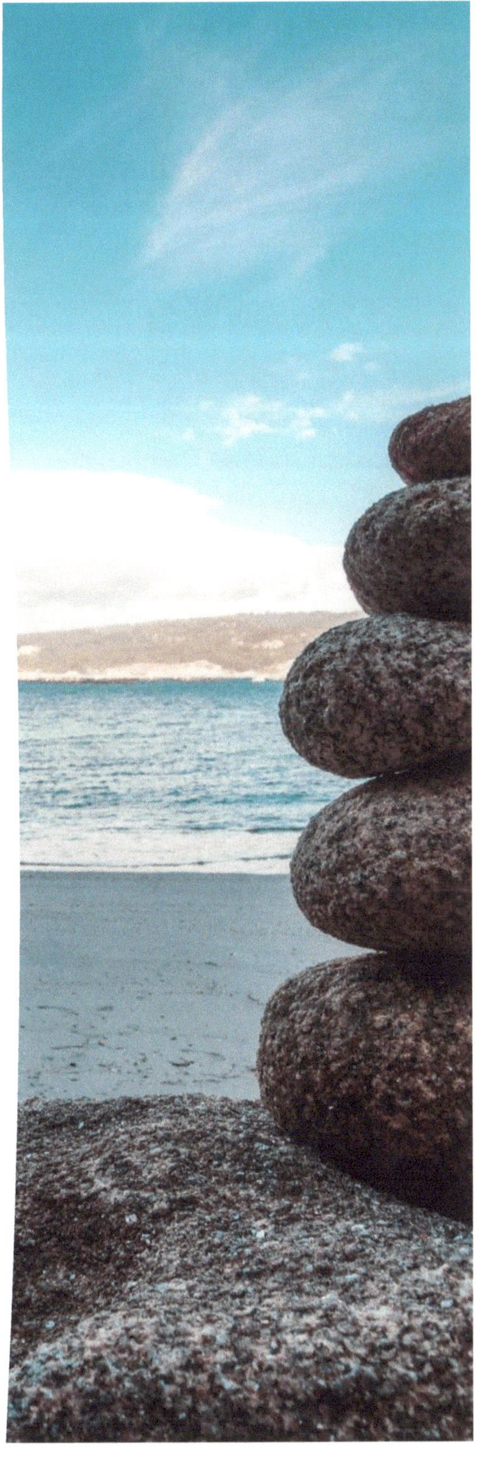

Facial Steam with Lavender Oil for Stress:
Ingredients: A few drops of lavender oil, hot water
Application: Add oil to hot water, inhale steam to relieve stress.

Cucumber Hair Treatment for Shine:
Ingredients: 1/2 cucumber, 1 tbsp olive oil
How to use: Puree cucumber, mix with olive oil, apply to hair, leave on for 30 minutes, rinse.

Blueberry Yogurt Face Mask for Glowing Skin:
Ingredients: Handful of fresh blueberries, 2 tbsp plain yoghurt
Application: Puree berries with yoghurt, apply to the face, leave on for 15 minutes, rinse.

Coconut Oil Sugar Body Scrub for Supple Skin:
Ingredients: 2 tbsp coconut oil, 1/2 cup sugar.
Application: Mix oil and sugar, apply to the skin as an exfoliant, massage in gently, rinse.

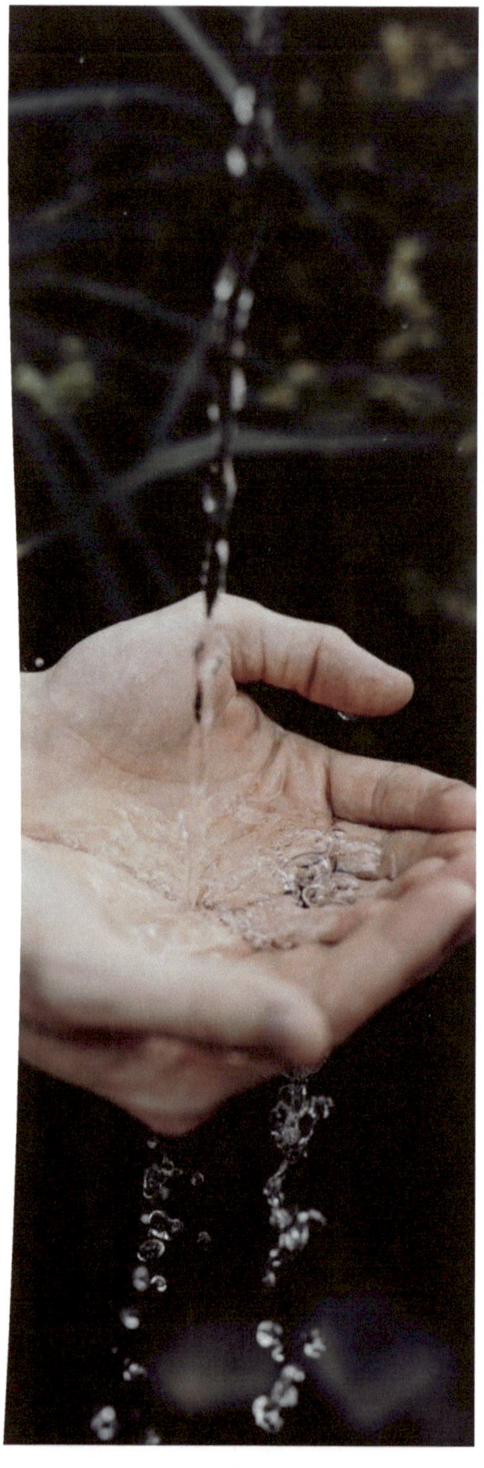

Avocado Honey Hair Mask for Shine:
Ingredients: 1/2 ripe avocado, 2 tbsp honey
How to use: Puree avocado, mix with honey, apply to hair, leave on for 30 minutes, rinse.

Lavender Lemon Oil Against Mosquitoes:
Ingredients: A few drops of lavender oil, a few drops of lemon oil, carrier oil (e.g. almond oil)
Application: Mix oils, apply to uncovered areas of skin to repel mosquitoes.

Apple Cider Vinegar Hair Conditioner for Shine & Dandruff:
Ingredients: 2 tbsp apple cider vinegar, 1 cup water
How to use: Use mixture as a final conditioner after shampooing to add shine and reduce dandruff.

Rosemary Garlic Oil for Nail Care:
Ingredients: A few sprigs of rosemary, 2 cloves of minced garlic, olive oil
How to use: Pickle rosemary and garlic in olive oil, strain, apply oil to nails to promote nail health.

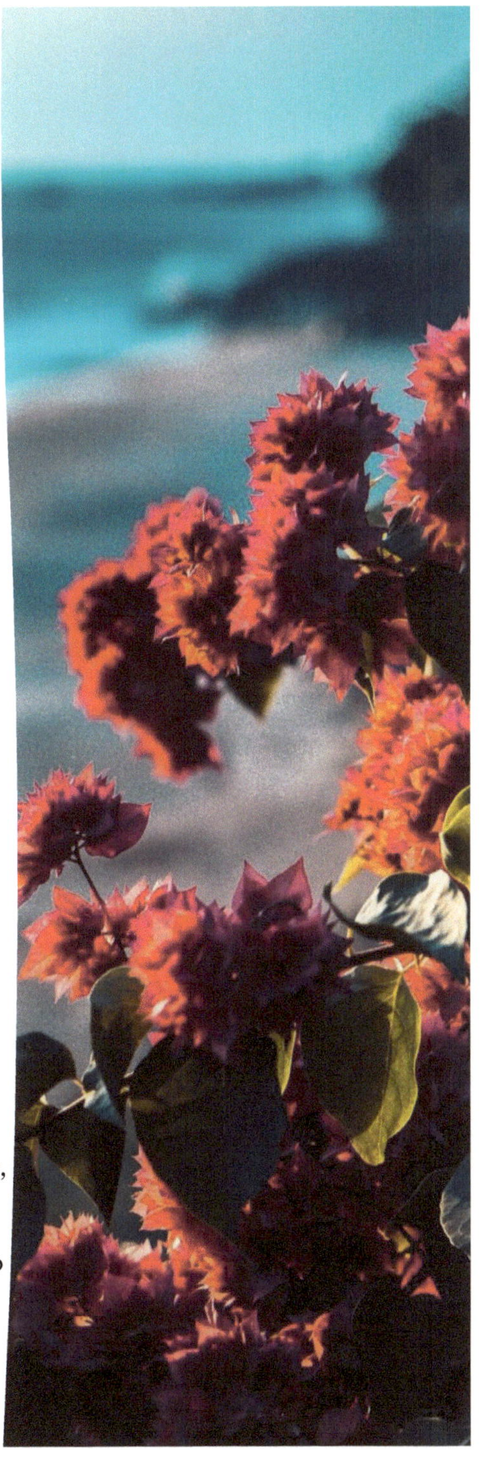

Pumpkin Honey Mask for Dry Skin:
Ingredients: 2 tbsp pumpkin puree, 1 tbsp honey
How to use: Apply mixture to the face, leave on for 20 minutes, rinse.

Mango Sugar Body Scrub for Soft Skin:
Ingredients: 1/2 ripe mango, 2 tbsp sugar
Application: Puree the mango, mix with sugar, use as a body scrub, rinse.

Parsley Hair Treatment for Hair Loss:
Ingredients: A handful of fresh parsley, 2 tbsp olive oil
How to use: Pickle parsley in olive oil, strain, massage oil onto the scalp to counteract hair loss.

Tea Tree Oil Toothpaste for Oral Hygiene:
Ingredients: 1 tsp coconut oil, 1 tsp baking powder, a few drops of tea tree oil
How to use: Mix ingredients, use as toothpaste to support oral hygiene.

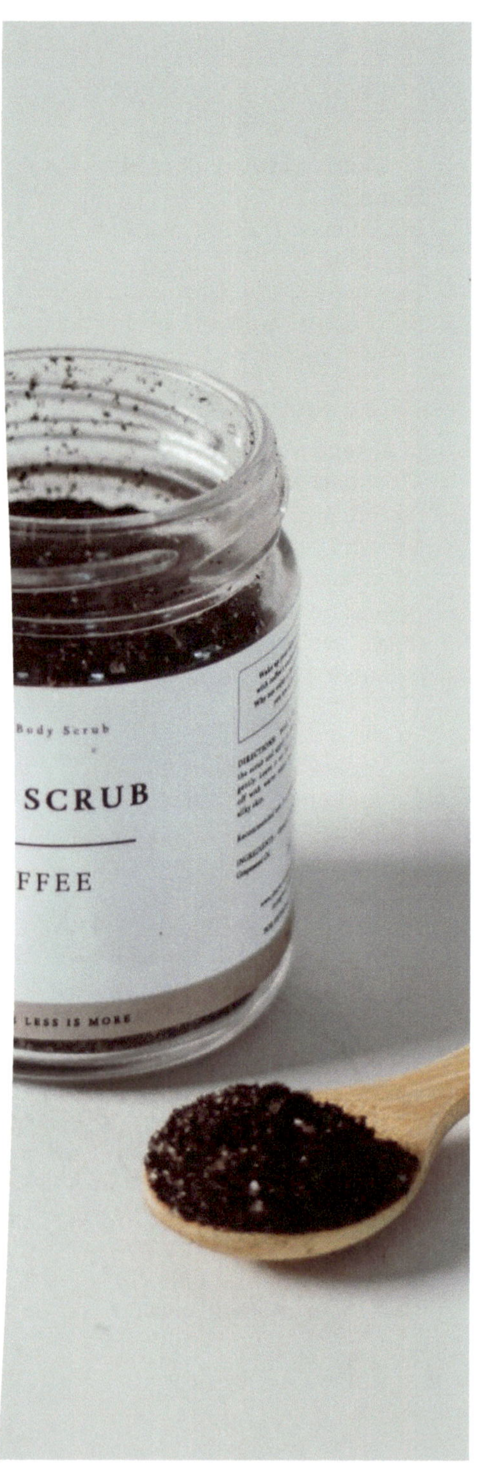

Rice Water for Skin Care:
Ingredients: 1/2 cup rice, water
Application: Boil rice, strain water, allow to cool, use as a facial toner.

Blueberry Yogurt Mask for Glowing Skin:
Ingredients: Handful of fresh blueberries, 2 tbsp plain yoghurt
Application: Puree berries with yoghurt, apply to the face, leave on for 15 minutes, rinse.

Charcoal Toothpaste for White Teeth:
Ingredients: 1 tsp activated charcoal powder, 1 tsp coconut oil
Application: Mix powder and oil, put on the toothbrush, brush your teeth, rinse.

Salt & Honey Gargle Solution for Sore Throat:
Ingredients: 1 tsp salt, 1 tsp honey, 1 cup warm water
How to use: Gargle mixture to relieve sore throat.

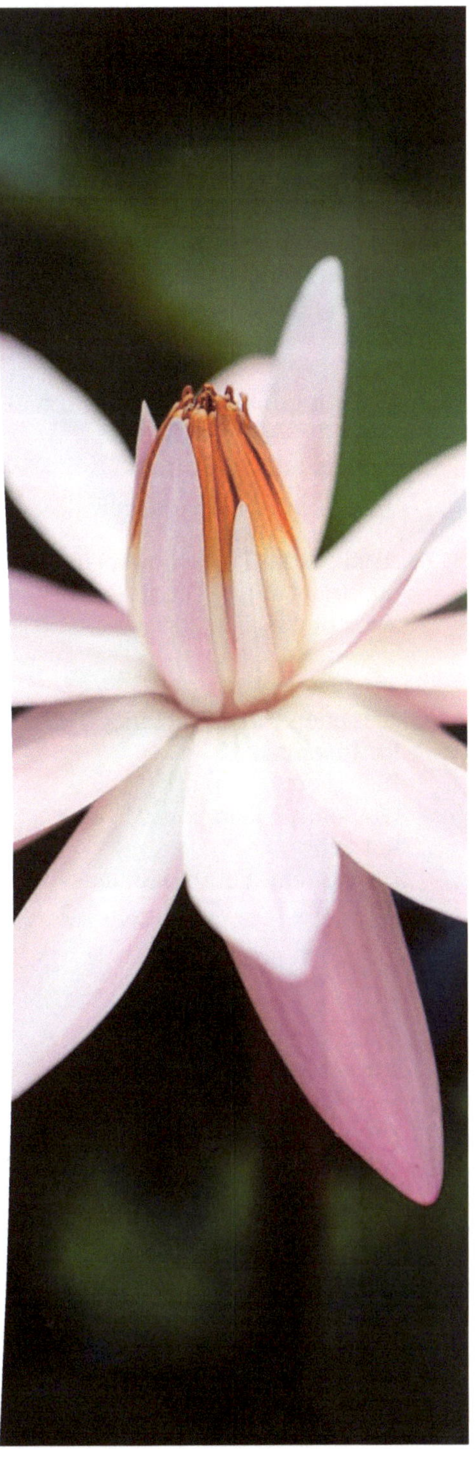

**Green Tea for Hair
Conditioner:**
Ingredients: 2 green tea bags, 1
cup of hot water
Application: Steep tea bags in
hot water, allow to cool, use as a
hair conditioner.

**Chamomile ointment for dry
skin:**
Ingredients: 2 tsp dried
chamomile flowers, 1/4 cup
coconut oil
Application: Pickle flowers in
oil, strain, apply ointment to dry
areas of the skin.

**Linden Blossom Honey Tea
for Insomnia:**
Ingredients: 1 tsp dried lime
blossoms, 1 tbsp honey, 1 cup
hot water
Application: Pour hot water
over flowers, add honey, drink
before going to bed.

**Lemon balm bath for
stress:**
Ingredients: Handful of fresh
lemon balm, hot water
Application: Infuse leaves in hot
water, add to bath water to
relieve stress.

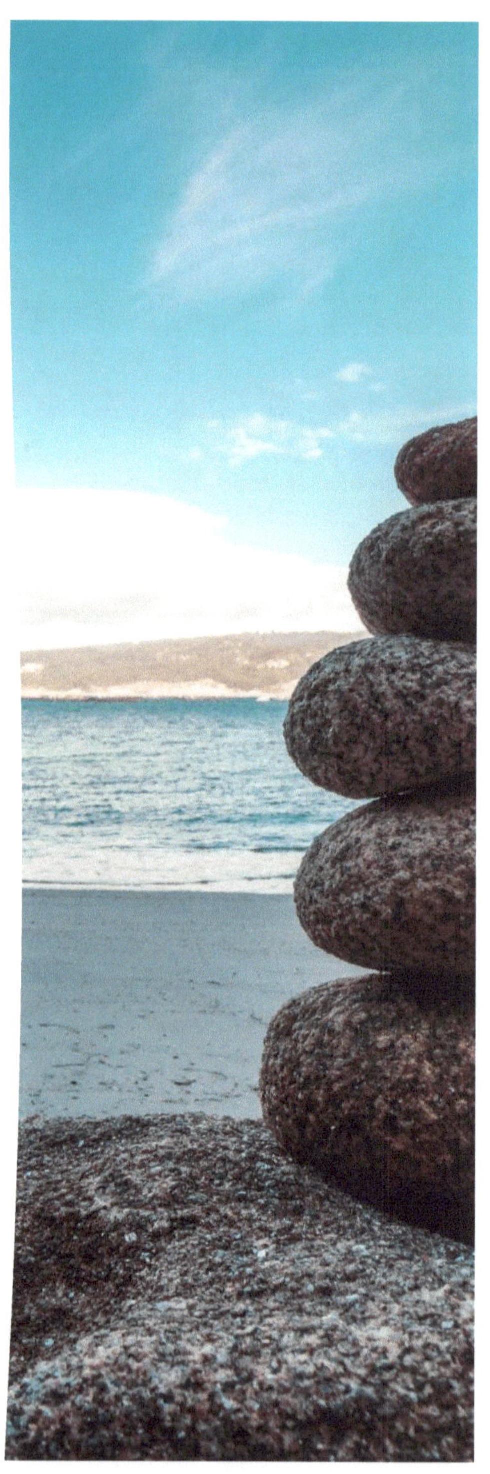

Garlic Honey Syrup for Cold:
Ingredients: 3 cloves of garlic, 2 tbsp honey
Application: Squeeze garlic, mix with honey, take syrup for colds.

Pineapple Honey Facial Scrub:
Ingredients: 2 tbsp fresh pineapple juice, 1 tbsp honey
How to use: Mix ingredients, apply to the face, massage gently, rinse.

Rosemary Lemon Hair Conditioner for Shine:
Ingredients: A few sprigs of rosemary, juice of one lemon, 2 cups of water
Application: Boil rosemary in water, allow to cool, mix with lemon juice, use as a hair conditioner.

Grapefruit hair mask for dandruff:
Ingredients: juice of half a grapefruit, 2 tbsp olive oil
How to use: Mix ingredients, apply to scalp, leave on for 20 minutes, rinse.

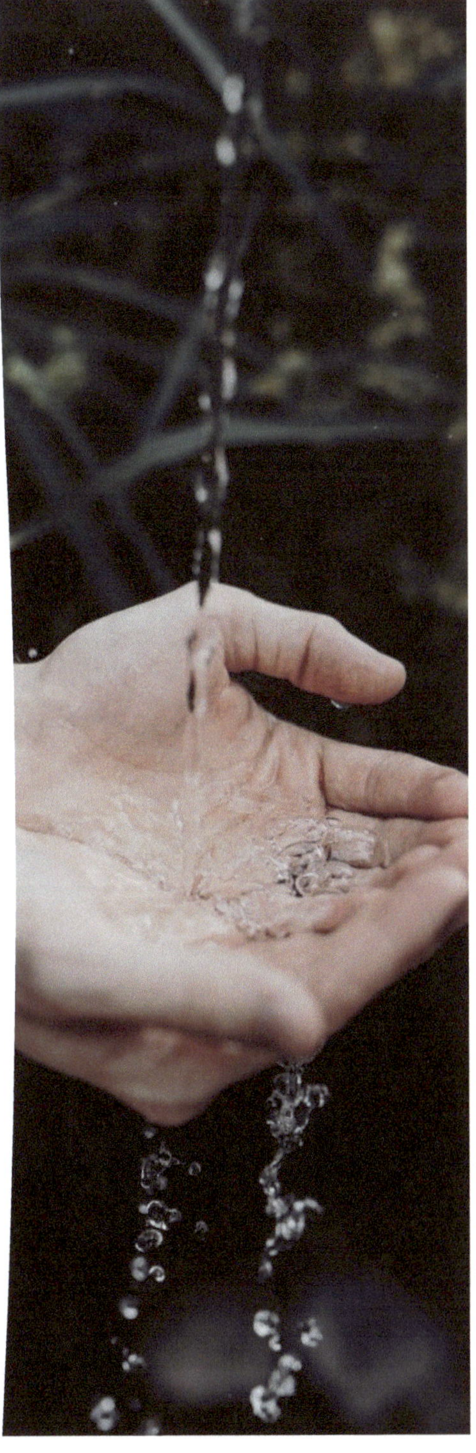

Lavender baths for insomnia:
Ingredients: A few drops of lavender oil, warm bath water
Application: Add oil to the bath water, bathe before going to bed to relieve sleep disturbances.

Basil Honey Face Scrub:
Ingredients: Handful of fresh basil leaves, 1 tbsp honey, 2 tbsp sugar
How to use: Mix ingredients, apply to the face, massage gently, rinse.

Cinnamon Honey Mask for Glowing Skin:
Ingredients: 1 tsp cinnamon, 1 tbsp honey
How to use: Apply mixture to face, leave on for 15 minutes, rinse.

St. John's wort tea against nervous restlessness:
Ingredients: 1 tsp dried St. John's wort flowers, 1 cup hot water
Application: Pour hot water over the flowers, strain, drink tea to relieve nervous restlessness.

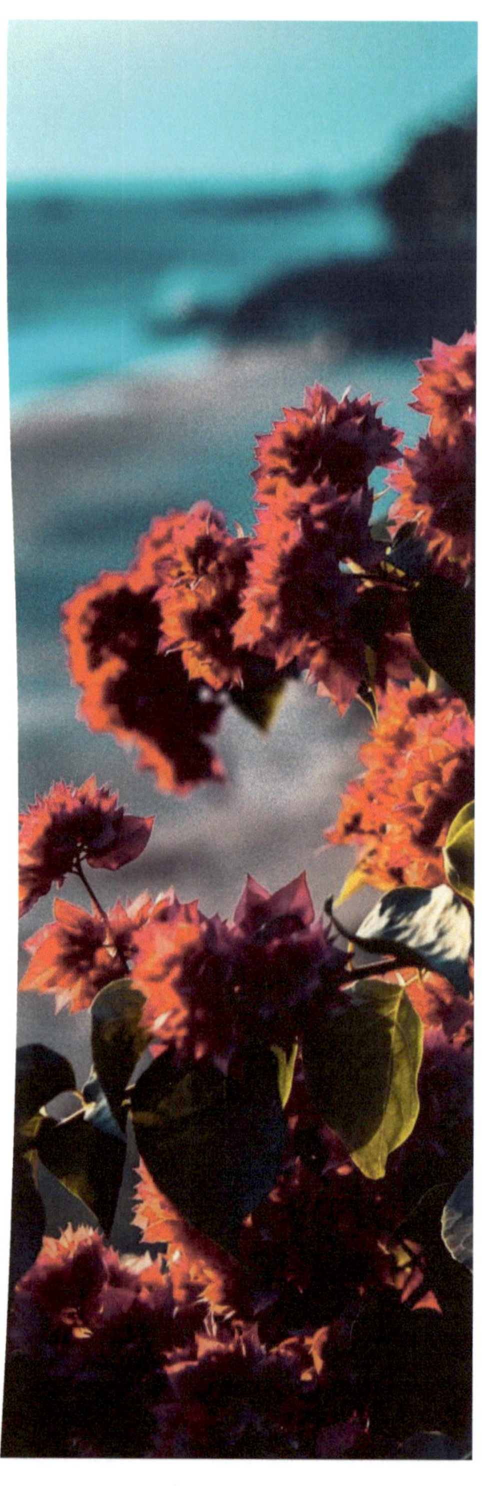

**Almond Oil Eye Compress
for Dryness:**
Ingredients: Almond oil, sterile
compress
Application: Soak compress in
almond oil, place on closed
eyes to relieve dryness.

**Chamomile Hair
Conditioner for Shine:**
Ingredients: 2 chamomile tea
bags, 2 cups hot water
Application: Steep tea bags in
hot water, allow to cool, use as a
hair conditioner.

**Avocado Honey Facial
Scrub:**
Ingredients: 1/2 ripe avocado, 2
tbsp honey, 1 tbsp sugar
Application: Puree the avocado,
mix with honey and sugar, apply
as a scrub, rinse.

**Yogurt Turmeric Mask for
Glowing Skin:**
Ingredients: 1 tsp turmeric
powder, 2 tbsp plain yoghurt
How to use: Apply mixture to
face, leave on for 15 minutes,
rinse.

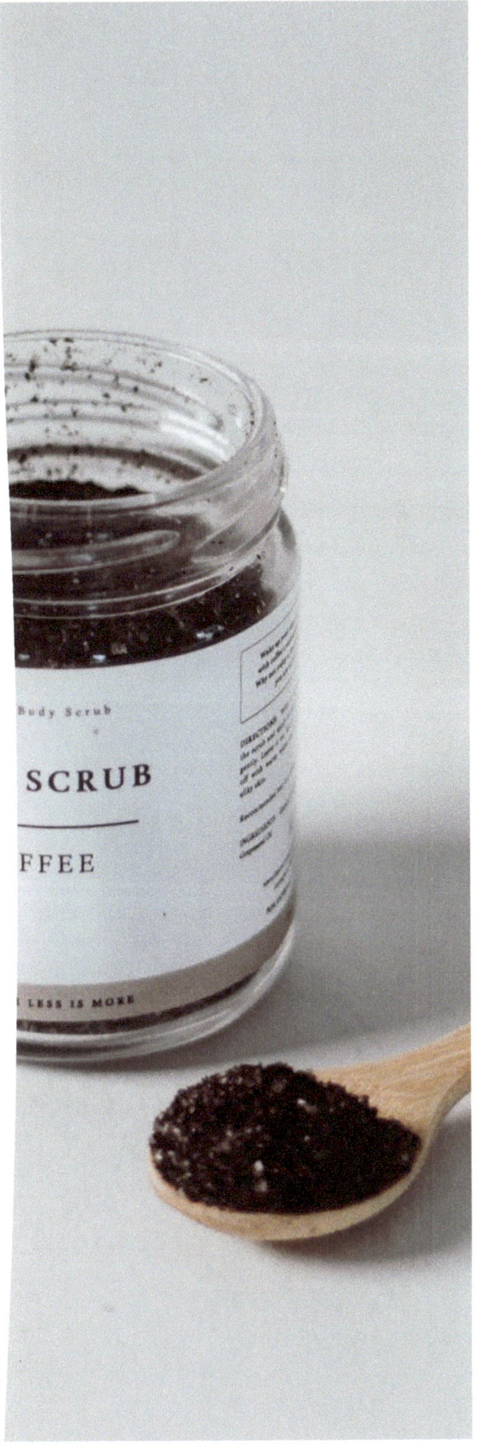

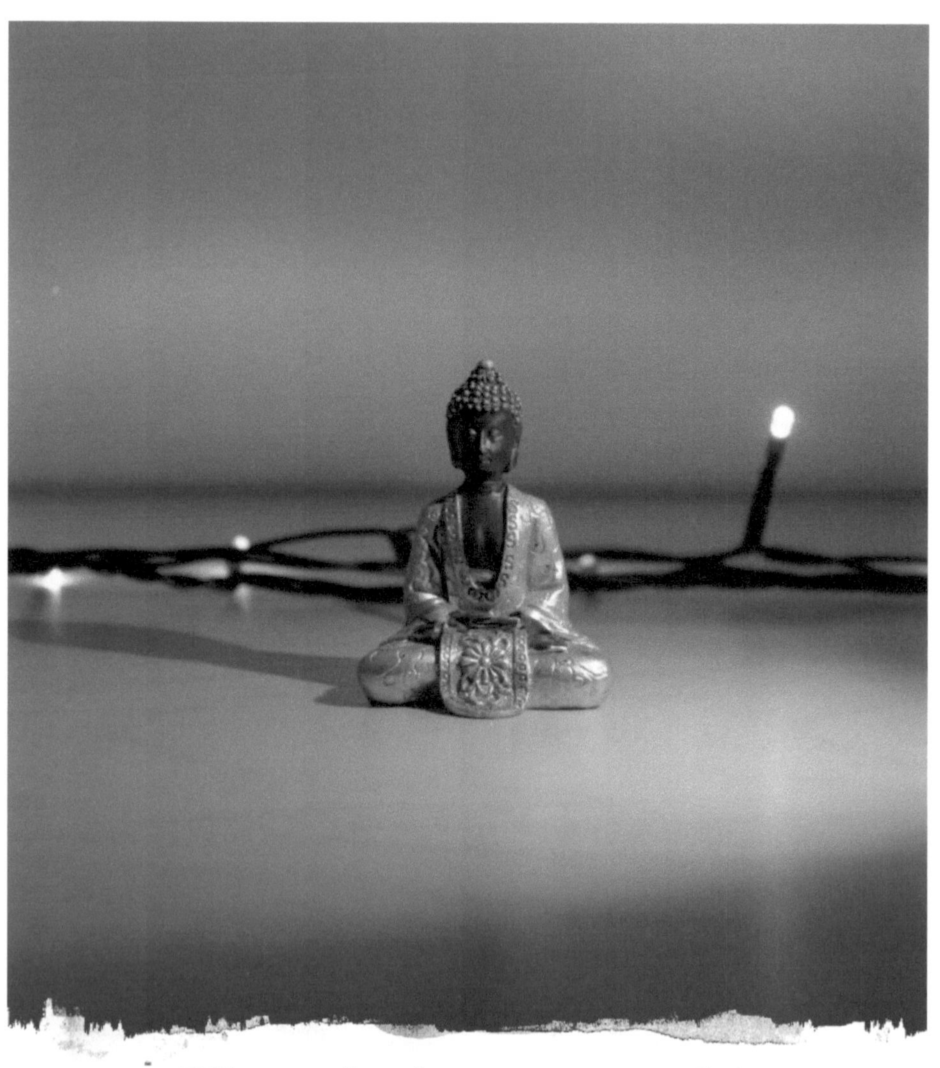

We say thank you very much !

"Traveling well is **better** than arriving." – Buddha